How to Ir
Doctor-Patient
Connection

Using psychology to optimize
healthcare interactions

Doctors and patients have a role in connecting with each other. This book integrates the perspective of a doctor and the view from the patient side, focusing on the use of cognitive habits of observing, listening, and emotional logic toward the goal of good medicine for every patient who needs it. The book is easy to read with clear divisions; gray pages have supplemental information, and black pages have practical applications that can be used in daily life to form strong habits that can be applied to healthcare encounters. Carefully learning to habitually use your perceptions to monitor the right data, make accurate decisions, and deliver precise messages will improve doctor-patient connection.

Christine J. Ko, MD is a Professor of Dermatology and Pathology at Yale University. She studied at Princeton University and New York University School of Medicine. She has published extensively in academic journals.

First published 2022
by Routledge
605 Third Avenue, New York, NY 10158

and by Routledge
2 Park Square, Milton Park, Abingdon, Oxon, OX14 4RN

Routledge is an imprint of the Taylor & Francis Group, an informa business

Library of Congress Cataloging-in-Publication Data
A catalog record for this title has been requested

ISBN: 978-0-367-76945-1 (hbk)
ISBN: 978-0-367-76947-5 (pbk)
ISBN: 978-1-003-16906-2 (ebk)

DOI: 10.4324/9781003169062

Publisher's note: This book has been prepared from camera-ready copy provided by the authors.

Typeset in Myriad Pro by Saheran Shoukat

To Susan
umuntu ngumuntu ngabantu

ACKNOWLEDGEMENTS

Thank you to Lucy Kennedy and her team at Routledge and Taylor & Francis (including Matthew Bickerton and Danielle Dyal) for believing in this book.

Many thanks to all the readers who were willing to look at multiple different drafts, including Susan Ko, PhD, David Caruso, PhD, Adam M Grant, PhD, William Vance, PhD, Pat Croskerry, MD PhD, Mark Abdelmalek, MD, Carly B. Dierkhising, PhD, Saeromi Kim, PhD, Belinda Tan, MD PhD, Jennifer McNiff, MD, J. Thomas Roland Jr, MD, Saul Weiner, MD, Neil Prose, MD, Flo Selfman, Joe Rusko, Victor Montori, MD, Randi Epstein, MD MPH, Anna Reisman, MD, Janice Harper, PhD, Janet Hafler, PhD, and Lisa Tener. Special mention to Susan Ko, PhD, who willingly read more drafts than anyone can imagine; and David Caruso, PhD, who graced me with his expertise in emotional intelligence with wonderful suggestions, edits, and comments for multiple chapters and particularly Chapters 9 and 10. Any errors or omissions are solely my responsibility.

I also give credit to Sammy Oh, Saheran Shoukat, Dylan Whang, and Owen Whang for their wonderful design abilities, opinions, and advice.

Bringing a book to publication requires support, and these individuals provided much needed encouragement along the way, including Julie Silver, MD, Zoe Chance, Suzanne Staszak-Silva, Andrew Kinney, Jennifer Chen Tran, and Yasmine Ali, MD.

Learning to be a good doctor is a work-in-progress for me, and deep appreciation to all of my patients, my teachers, and mentors; some of the latter are mentioned by name in the text, with their permission; others are not but are no less important, including Richard Edelson, MD, David Leffell, MD, Leonard Milstone, MD, Antonio Subtil Deoliveira, MD, MBA, Scott Binder, MD, Gary Cole, MD, Edward Jeffes III, MD, PhD, Vandana Nanda, MD, Kenneth Linden, MD, PhD, M. Joy Rico, MD, and Robert Modlin, MD.

Last but not least, thank you to my family and especially my two children, who teach me every day about what can be possible.

Table of Contents

LEARNING FROM FAILURE: MY OWN EXPERIENCE OF DOCTOR-PATIENT CONNECTION

"Do not fear mistakes. You will know failure. Continue to reach out."
— Benjamin Franklin, American Polymath

On paper, I have achieved success as a faculty member at Yale, handling a full-time clinical practice, teaching in various situations locally and nationally, and having objective evidence of scholarly activity. Despite that, this book developed because I failed spectacularly. One of my new patients refused to see me again because she felt that I am not thorough with my total body skin examination, one of the main things I do as a clinical dermatologist. The icing on the cake is that I personally know this patient, and when I asked her to give me another chance, she felt strongly enough about her experience that she politely refused. *She was not willing to step into my examination room ever again.*

Her perception is that I missed a skin cancer that was growing in the center of her face. She had pointed it out to me at the end of the visit as I was about to leave the room, asking me if I had noted it. *Yes,* I said, *I am not concerned about that. I don't think it is skin cancer. You know where to find me* (remember that we knew each other!), *and we can watch it.* My words did not reassure her, and we mutually decided to biopsy it right then and there – remove it and send it to the lab for a diagnosis which ended up being an early "actinic keratosis", not a skin cancer but a precancer. Not all precancers need to be treated or removed as not all progress to skin cancer and some even disappear without any treatment. The human body is amazing! I gave her this good news, and it was only later that she told me that the biopsy results didn't change things – she still didn't feel comfortable having me as her doctor.

Imagine if all of my patients felt this way – there would be no one for me to see in my clinic – the patient's perception of his/her experience of my doctoring absolutely matters. I thought and felt I had given the patient good medical care, but her perception was the opposite. I had failed.

ABOUT ME

Before we go further, a little background on me. I am a physician, a Professor of Dermatology and Pathology at Yale University. I am married, and together my husband and I are the sometimes harried parents of two children, a teenage daughter with typical hearing and a preteen son who is deaf, has bilateral cochlear implants, and achieved age-matched spoken language by age six.[1] As a daughter of two Korean immigrants, I was born in

---

[1] As a quick introduction, if you are not aware of what this means – cochlear implants are not the same as hearing aids. Hearing aids amplify sound; cochlear implants send electrical impulses encoding sound to the brain. Cochlear implants require surgery, either on one side alone (unilateral) or both ears (bilateral); they have an internally implanted component and an external electronic device that requires programming, has batteries, and is not worn while sleeping.

the melting pot of the United States but spent much of my childhood in my supposed motherland of South Korea (attending a private American school), experiencing cultural and language barriers with my sister as "foreigners", given English is our first and native language, while always being told that Korean is our "mother tongue" (and literally our mother's first and native language). I work full-time outside of the home as well as a good amount inside the home, and I am also lucky to have hired someone reliable to help keep my home life on track. At work, I am a "clinician-educator", which is a good job description – I examine patients' skin in clinic, read microscopic slides of skin biopsies, and teach visual recognition, just not at a chalkboard. I teach to increase the dermatology and dermatopathology knowledge of my patients, trainees, and other physicians, one-to-one, in groups, and remotely through books, lectures, and medical articles. As most parents know, home life with young kids means you are hardly ever alone (even the privacy of the bathroom is not sacred!), and my relationships at work, home, and any space in between can be relentless. As an introvert, I find relationships hard, but I still need them. Through teaching my son language, my work experience with visual perception (I spend at least 4 hours each work day making diagnoses based on what I see) melded with what I began learning of auditory and emotional perception to form relevant habits that helped me connect with not only my son but also my patients.

THE DUNNING-KRUGER EFFECT

Focusing on auditory perception with my son created a deep connection between us, and this connection included my daughter as well given that she actively participated in much of what we did. The strong bond that grew from the auditory therapy we did as a family demonstrated to me that I can actively improve my ability to connect. Meanwhile, prior to embarking on the long road of teaching my son speech and language, I am pretty sure that I would have predicted that I could easily connect with my own children. Through the process of intense speech and language therapy with my son, I learned that my prediction would have been a classic example of "being unskilled and unaware". Such a false sense of competence, particularly when unskilled, is pervasive among all human beings and even has a name – it is called the Dunning-Kruger effect. The Dunning-Kruger effect affects us all and may be at least partially responsible for my failure with the patient I described. Doctors may be poor diagnosticians or communicators but think that they are very skilled. Patients and family members may not fully understand a healthcare diagnosis; despite this deficiency, they may believe or pretend that total comprehension is there.

Knowing that you can be affected by the effect of misperceived competence, you can take extra care to more fully evaluate what is happening during a healthcare interaction through carefully examining what is seen, heard, and felt. You will be less prone to missing or misinterpreting information. You can double-check any conclusions you come to and create healthier relationships that will benefit communication, medical diagnosis, and treatment plans. This simply involves thinking about what you see, hear, and feel.

Returning to my failure with my own patient and her negative perception of our interaction, the experience made me confront my being "unskilled and unaware" in my doctor-patient relationships. I realized I wanted to do better.

THE GOOD NEWS

While moment-to-moment your brain can process 50,000 times the amount of information that is stored in the Library of Congress, you are rightly limited in perception and attention to avoid being buried by all that data. Fortunately, you can expand your visual, auditory, and emotional awareness by increasing connectivity within the brain, by grouping what you see, hear, and feel into one cohesive unit rather than multiple, disparate elements. You learn to group through practice and tiny adjustments that become second nature, similar to when you first learn to read or drive. For reading, children learn letters, sounds, phonics. They learn syllables, phrases, sentences. They learn to recognize words by sight, by sound, and even by their emotional underpinnings. Right now, you are reading without parsing every letter or syllable. In learning to drive, initially, the complex interplay of visual (e.g. the car itself, vehicles around you, traffic signals), auditory (e.g. the driving instructor, the car signals, ambient noise), and emotional stimulation (e.g. nervousness, excitement, surprise) can be overwhelming. Eventually, you can drive somewhere familiar and hardly remember how you got there. Cognitive habits generate automaticity; you become able to read or drive without consciously thinking about every step or stimulus. The cacophony of the experience becomes easy. And the good news is, if you know how to read or drive, you already have created the metaperceptive habits that this book addresses. Those same habits just need to be applied to the doctor-patient interaction.

THE GOAL OF THIS BOOK

Metaperception can create concrete habits. You are already using metaperceptive habits as you read this without thinking about the act of reading. Given the constraints on time that doctors and patients face, channeling habit is a way to create ease and multiply the time spent together. Thinking about what you see, hear, and feel is the start of more efficient chunking of visual, auditory, and emotional data. Chunking data will eventuate, over time, into habits of consistently observing more, listening better, and reacting logically; and these habits will improve doctor-patient connection.

AN IDEAL PATIENT-DOCTOR CONNECTION

Dr. J. Thomas Roland says to me, *Let us help you shoulder this burden. You are not alone.*

These two sentences continue to linger in my head, even now, close to eight years after I first heard them. They were an expression of empathy, gifted to me by the doctor that we chose as the cochlear implant surgeon for my then two-year-old son.

Dr. Roland was the first healthcare professional who said anything of that nature to me in the initial, scary three months after my son was diagnosed (too late) at age two with profound deafness. I felt as though he saw me, and he saw my son. I felt as though my son and I mattered; *whatever the outcome,* he would be a bulwark against an unpredictable storm. He would bear witness.

The words may have affected me more because, if you had asked me, I would have said it wasn't important if the doctor actually cared about my son. I would have said that I just wanted the best doctor, the best surgeon, the best team. I chose Dr. Roland because my research indicated that he was technically excellent, one of the best cochlear implant surgeons in the world, based on reputation, experience, and number of surgeries (by chance, he happened to be at my *alma mater*, and I did some private digging, asking several former classmates if they had worked with him in the operating room). The choice of surgeon was critical to me because the risks of surgery cast a heavy, dark shadow over the process; not only could the cochlear implants be ineffective for my son's particular diagnosis, the process of implantation would destroy any native function of the cochlea, there were risks of meningitis and facial paralysis, and I had been reading that the Deaf community likened cochlear implantation of babies and toddlers to genital mutilation (the latter being absolutely horrifying to me and not something I would ever want to consider as an option for either of my children).

I'm not sure who our surgeon would have been, had Dr. Roland not said those words to me, had he not presented me with such warmth and comfort, had he not literally picked up my curious son (who was touching everything in the examination room), enfolding him with a genuine smile. His reputation for technical expertise probably would have made him our first choice no matter what. And for such a superlative surgeon to also seem to recognize my

"Let us help you shoulder this burden. You are not alone."

— J. Thomas Roland, MD

son's humanity – it was a priceless gift, one I hadn't imagined before receiving.

How was he so successful at giving me comfort while in contrast my own doctoring and past experiences were somewhat cold, unemotional, and detached? It was a combination of my own stress, my openness and honesty, and his response to me. I believe he saw my future hopes and fears, he listened to my worries, he felt the diagnostic delay that I was trying to make up for. He saw me, heard me, and understood my emotions with precision and accuracy, responding in a situationally appropriate manner that was, in the moment, flawless. He was also the third surgeon that I took my son to see, so I had already had "practice" in meeting a surgeon, interacting, and being given a treatment plan. I met him fully prepared and conscious of what I wanted to ask.

OVERVIEW

Here is an overview of the book. I will tell you about the background behind the importance of doctor-patient connection (relationship-centered care) in **Chapter 1**. **Chapter 2** covers metacognition, thinking about how we think, specifically as it relates to how doctors and patients interact. **Chapters 3** and **4** address metacognition in diagnosis and communication in healthcare. A broad overview of three major cognitive intelligences as used to form visual, auditory, and emotional habits using relevant data is in **Chapters 5 to 10. Chapter 11** brings everything together. The main text in each chapter is concise and divided into sections, with key information in the subsection on doctor-patient connection. Supplemental anecdotes and text that probe deeper to reinforce certain concepts are on pages with **gray shading**. Practical applications in daily life will grow stronger habits, and suggested exercises on **black-shaded pages** relate to applying the information directly back to forming habits toward doctor-patient connection in your own healthcare encounters.

EYE COLOR

For a period of time, I focused on noting the eye color of my patients within the first moments of walking into a patient room – I realized it helped me connect as it forced me to gaze directly at the patient's face, making eye contact. Eye contact helps build trust between doctor and patient, and it helped me establish rapport. After focusing on eye color for a couple of weeks, I no longer had to think about it – the color of a patient's eyes became something I noticed almost immediately as I greeted them, without my consciously having to think about it. Visual perception of eye color is now habit for me, and personally, it helps me to remember to try to see the world from the patient's perspective. This simple technique may not work for everyone, and the exercises at the end of each chapter can help you pinpoint something that is most relevant to your own healthcare encounters.

This book has a good amount of focus on everyday tasks, particularly in the suggested practical applications, because true change happens when you use habits in your personal life and allow them to spill over into your work life. Medical students and seasoned physicians alike often hold patients at arms-length, not speaking to patients as they would to "real people". Polite, scared, or reticent patients may not be fully able to share in what can feel like an inappropriately intrusive medical encounter, especially on meeting a doctor for the first time. Healthcare interactions are often put in their own special category of communication. But connecting between doctor and patient should not be any different than establishing a relationship with another person who matters, and thinking about what you see, hear, and feel provides tools to do this.

Focusing on relationship-centered care for doctor-patient connection has changed me. As a doctor, I had plenty of experience learning about diseases, medical advances, and treatments, but patient care is more than just medical diagnosis. As a shy introvert, I didn't have a reliable method to approach the patient encounter beyond standard medical diagnosis, treatment, and planning. Despite having had a certain amount of healthcare exposure from the patient side (I had already had one in-hospital delivery with all the associated prenatal care), I didn't have a reliable method to optimize healthcare from the patient side, either, in terms of advocating for myself or my children. In essence, I was connecting with my patients and my family's doctors through luck; if it happened, wonderful, and if it didn't, well... I could try harder next time.

I have now realized that rather than pushing myself to do more in already busy medical visits, I can better connect in doctor-patient interactions by channeling metacognitive habits. Habits make things easy and ultimately save time. While this book is primarily directed at physicians because they interact with patients often daily, almost every physician also is a patient, at one point or another. A relationship is a two-way street, and patients interested in better healthcare utilization can benefit from reading about how doctors think and what can help to establish a good doctor-patient connection and true relationship-centered care. Healthcare can be too important to trust random chance, and habitually using what you see, hear, and feel provides a reliable, structured approach for good medicine.

KEY CONCEPTS
Relationship-centered care

In any patient-physician interaction, there are two sides, two perceptions, two realities. I wouldn't say that the patient is always right, but as a doctor I do know that, much to my chagrin, the doctor is not always right, either! Because of this, relationship-centered care is important – physicians are the medical experts in the room, and patients are experts of their own experience, needs, and concerns.

In relationship-centered care, doctors and patients connect and share their specific expertise; they are stronger for navigating healthcare together. There is no one-size fits all model; a given patient-physician interaction is unique. Read the previous section on **An Ideal Patient-Doctor Connection** for a positive example of my own experience of relationship-centered care as the mother of a patient.

"Physician flexibility is the skill necessary to address variation in patient preference."
— Richard Frankel, PhD
Professor of Medicine

Metacognition

Metacognition simply is thinking about your thinking. Dr. Daniel Kahneman, a Nobel-prize winning psychologist, has coined the terms, "System 1" and "System 2", to refer to your major thinking patterns. "System 1" is fast thinking, your instinctive response, your gut "feeling". "System 2" is slow thinking, careful, logical, more conscious. Neither System truly exists, they are semantic markers. Neither System is better than the other, and both can lead to errors in your thinking.

Metaperception

"Meta"-ness has entered our thinking and has seeped into popular wisdom. There are meta-data, meta-analysis, and meta-skills. Metaperception is defined here as thinking about what you see, hear, and feel to optimize observation, listening, and emotional processing. Arguably, perception is a form of cognition, in which case, metaperception can be considered a type of metacognition.

> "The reality we perceive, feel, see and hear is influenced by the constructive processes of the brain as well as by the cues that impinge upon it."
> — Merlin Wittrock, PhD, Educational Psychologist

FURTHER READING

5 A false sense of competence, particularly when unskilled, is pervasive...Kruger J, et al. Unskilled and unaware of it: How difficulties in recognizing one's own incompetence lead to inflated self-assessments. *J Personal Soc Psychol* 1999;77:1121-1134.

7 Process 50,000 times the amount of information...Marois R, et al. Capacity limits of information processing in the brain. *Trends in Cognitive Sciences* 2005;9:296-305.

7 You are rightly limited in perception and attention...Driver J, et al. Perceptual awareness and its loss in unilateral neglect and extinction. *Cognition* 2011;79:39.

7 Similar to when you first learn to read or drive... Duhigg, Charles. *The Power Of Habit: Why We Do What We Do In Life And Business.* New York: Random House, 2012.

7 Eventually, you can drive somewhere familiar and hardly remember how you got there... Kahneman D. *Thinking, Fast and Slow.* New York: Farrar, Straus and Giroux, 2011.

11 And for such a superlative surgeon to also have empathy for me...Laidlaw TS, et al. What makes a physician an exemplary communicator with patients? *Patient Educ Couns* 2007;68:153-160.

13 Eye contact helps build trust between doctor and patient...Tate P, Frame F. *The Doctor's Communication Handbook,* 8th edition. Boca Raton: CRC Press, 2019;1-142.

14 Patient care is more than just medical diagnosis...Hojat M, et al. Physicians' empathy and clinical outcomes for diabetic patients. *Acad Med* 2011;86:359-364.

16 Because of this, relationship-centered care is important...Beach MC and Inui T. Relationship-centered care. A constructive reframing. *J Gen Intern Med* 2006;21 Suppl 1:S3-8.

16 Experts of their own experience, needs, and concerns...Gavin F. The risks of equating 'lived experience' with patient expertise. *Healthy Debate: Opinions.* 2019.

17 Dr. Daniel Kahneman, a Nobel-prize winning psychologist, has coined the terms, "System 1" and "System 2",...Kahneman D. *Thinking, Fast and Slow*. New York: Farrar, Straus and Giroux, 2011.

1 A DOCTOR'S DOCTOR: SHOWING HUMANITY

"…to the extent that you can, *err in the direction of kindness.*"
— George Saunders, American Writer, Syracuse University 2013 Commencement Address

I am silently crying, my eyes and cheeks damp, teardrops collecting on my jawline to drip and pepper my shirt with small, dark polka dots. I sit, feeling frozen, the future a yawning black hole given today's revelation that my two-year-old son is profoundly deaf, memories from the past surfacing like perfectly lined-up dominoes falling, falling, falling in sync.

As a newborn, you remain peacefully sleeping without even a twitch as your three-year-old sister and her friend noisily enter the family room, giggling and chattering loudly, completely oblivious of your presence in the baby recliner. In your dream world, you are oblivious, too.

As a nine-month-old, you are once again napping, this time in your crib, when I accidentally release the doorknob so that it clicks, suddenly and loudly, sounding like a shotgun in the silent oasis of your room. You don't stir, and I am relieved that I didn't wake you, for an instant, before I instinctively know that your lack of response is not typical. Doctors tell me I am wrong.

As a twelve-month-old, you are busy, busy, busy; too busy to listen to me, I suppose. You play with blocks or whatever else catches your fancy, absorbed with them, ignoring my words. Everything goes in your mouth. Anything you can touch, you grab. Something new catches your eye, and you are off to explore. I take you to the doctor again, and once again I am told you have normal hearing; there is nothing wrong according to the doctor.

As a 15-month-old, you still have no words. Two lovely ladies from Birth to 3 come to our house and watch us play together. They hear my concerns about your language development and note that the doctors said your hearing is normal. They tell me that your language will blossom in the next couple of months. They tell me that they will "squeeze you in", just barely, into the Birth to 3 Program because you almost don't qualify – they think you are a typical boy; boys often have slightly delayed language. They will enroll you because they see my worry, and they tell me that you will be an "easy case" that leaves Birth to 3 successfully, with flying colors, in no time.

As an 18-month-old, you still have no words. One of the lovely ladies from Birth to 3 visits you in your daycare environment and accidentally drops her heavy binder. It crashes to the ground, demanding attention, and of the six toddlers in the room, you are the only one who blissfully ignores it. Five little heads swivel in unison toward the noise, and you remain focused; busy, busy, busy with your toy of the moment. The Birth to 3 teacher asks me if I am sure your hearing is normal. My heart simultaneously explodes and contracts because I haven't been sure of your hearing for over half your life. It is not a comfort that someone else is finally concerned.

As a 22-month-old, you are still in an anesthesia-induced sleep as I process what the doctor has just told me. *You are profoundly deaf. Your hearing is not normal. Your newborn screening tests and the tests we had before were not the right tests to detect your rare diagnosis.*

The doctor knows I can hear her because she sees my tears. I know she sees them because she hands me a box of Kleenex. We don't connect because she cannot see how the dominoes just fell in my head, and I try to pay attention as she starts talking about fitting you for ear molds so you can get hearing aids. I keep it together to point out that she had just showed me a flat line. The hearing part of your brain had produced a flat line. I'm a doctor, but I had only seen such a flat line on heart monitors when the heart is dead. *Wasn't the flat line a sign that the hearing brain is dead?* The doctor hardly blinks as she says, *Yes.* Then why hearing aids? She launches into a discussion of the future. The hearing aids are unlikely to work, but that's what insurance requires as a first treatment step. As the hearing aids were unlikely to work, the next step might be cochlear implants. Insurance might not approve that. Anyway, with a flat line, cochlear implants probably wouldn't work either. *But you might want to try. Lots of decisions to make,* she pronounces almost cheerily. *Why not get the ear molds made today? That will save you a visit.*

My husband has to go back to work, and I leave the hospital with you sleeping in my arms. I pass the husband of Dr. Jean Bolognia, a valued mentor of mine, and somehow my brain tells me that my mentor, who is one of the best diagnosticians that I know, a "doctor's doctor", will be able to help me with this diagnosis. And she does, because when I confess to her a few hours later that I am still crying, and I really shouldn't be because deafness is not a fatal diagnosis, she gently admonishes me, *You're only crying because you are human.* I am only human.

HUMANITY

My mentor, who knows more dermatology than anyone that I know, is a superlative doctor because she also recognizes each person's humanity. In retrospect, it is obvious to me that I already had the diagnosis for my son, and I was not actually consulting her for an opinion on the medical diagnosis. When I called her, I would not say that I myself explicitly knew what I was asking of her, someone already firmly entrenched in my mind as a "doctor's doctor". Thinking of her in that way, I do partially mean that she can provide dermatologic care to another doctor, because she has an unparalleled medical knowledge base. She will know things that other doctors do not know. She can provide clarity and great management plans that might escape other excellent physicians. She is a doctor's doctor.

With the lens of time, I can see that I was unknowingly asking something else of her, which she wonderfully provided – she saw me, she heard me, and she felt my fear and anxiety. She understood me that day; in contrast, the doctor who gave me my son's diagnosis didn't even comment on my tears. Handing me a box of Kleenex could be a sign of caring, but with no acknowledgment of my feelings or the doctor's, it is hard to know what the diagnosing doctor felt. Instead, the doctor immediately focused on important next steps (which I don't deny are important, then and now). I believe that doctor cared, but there was no way of knowing; the diagnosis of deafness and *what to do about it* quickly swallowed everything else in the room.

My own emotions were clearly on display, to both the diagnosing doctor and my mentor. To the doctor who gave me the diagnosis of deafness, deafness seemed relatively routine, nothing for her to react to. Or even perhaps, not something she *should* react to, because then it might be too difficult for her to get through the day. To a certain extent, doctors may hold back from being involved because it may seem like it would be too draining to be deeply affected by every new patient diagnosis. In a similar vein, many patients, including me with my tears, do not discuss their emotional reactions in a healthcare visit. It did not necessarily have to take more than a minute for me or the doctor to verbally acknowledge my tears and perhaps take just a moment to process the diagnosis together and create comfort. But neither of us tried to connect in this way.

When doctors remain "professional" and patients try to remain "composed", it is harder to sense the other's private world. Because patients are the ones that may be facing a difficult diagnosis for the first time, doctors are potentially able to foresee a patient's needs, using information given by the patient to create the patient's experience, including conceivable fears and anxiety, through the doctor's prior experience, imagination, and mental imagery (see section on the importance of imagination). For example, interviews with parents of patients with chronic medical conditions indicate the importance of giving parents of young children with significant medical diagnoses a sense of hope, an imagined future that is different from the dark one that patients and family members may initially see due to lack of experience with a given medical diagnosis. Parents of young children in need of chronic medical care repeatedly emphasized the need for healthcare professions to apprehend "the contours of their lives, at least once, from the inside."

Coming back to the day of my son's diagnosis, I didn't know (and couldn't imagine) what I may have hoped to receive from the doctor until my mentor gave me exactly what I needed – someone to bear witness to my humanity. I think many patients, especially doctors when they take on the role of patients, encounter the coldness of a serious medical diagnosis when delivered divorced from acknowledgment of the human beings involved. Through my experience of getting the proper medical diagnosis for my son and then also feeling seen by my mentor, I sensed firsthand how a true doctor's doctor might address *both* the medical *and* the psychosocial aspect of a heavy diagnosis. This *how* is actually almost too simple – it involves just thinking about what you see, hear, and feel in a given interaction.

IMAGINATION AND MENTAL IMAGERY

Metaperception, thinking about what you see, hear, and feel, gives substance and form to using imagination and mental imagery to create someone's private personhood and humanity with accuracy and compassion. Unlike close friends or family members who we can generally see in their natural environments, a patient's daily, lived experience can only be imagined by the physician through

"…we listen not only with our ears, but with our eyes, mind, heart and imagination…"

— Carl Rogers, American Psychologist

seeing, hearing, and feeling during a healthcare interaction to construct an image of a given patient.

While not necessarily easy in each and every interaction, this type of imagination and mental imagery should not feel too unfamiliar, as you perform such mental imagery with the very image you hold of yourself – your own thoughts on what you see, hear, and feel about your own self – your own perspective of yourself may not fully match that of others or real-time changes. Dr. Maxwell Maltz was a facial plastic surgeon who was struck by the differing reactions of his patients to their altered appearance after plastic surgery. Only the minority of them changed their attitudes about themselves; the vast majority looked different but felt no different. Their perception of their appearances was the same; real-time physical changes ultimately had no bearing on their self-image. Dr. Maltz researched this curious phenomenon and suggested that your *mental image* of yourself is largely what drives your personality and who you think you are. Even the concrete physical characteristics as perceived by others or in a mirror are secondary and often not as relevant. Imagination (your perceived reality) is what you use for self-perception, and that same imagination can be used to perceive others. The doctor should ask, *Who is this patient in his/her own eyes?* The patient should ask, *Can the doctor truly see who I am?* It is important for doctors to think about this question, and patients can help doctors by being open and presenting themselves as accurately as possible.

THE TROUBLE WITH IMAGINATION

Understanding a patient's (or for that matter, anyone else's) private world is fraught with error. It is both amazingly easy and excruciatingly difficult – it is easy because you are used to interacting with people, and you know what it feels like to know friends and family well. It is difficult because the healthcare interaction is a proscribed relationship, often initially between two strangers, one of whom (generally the patient) may reveal deeply personal healthcare information in a first encounter that normally only very close friends or family would be privy to. Patients may be stressed or anxious, and doctors also may be anxious, either for personal reasons or due to the ever-more-present time pressure in healthcare. Connecting is also difficult because you've seen that emotions can run high between friends and among family members, and even close friendships and family are not immune to miscommunication, misinterpretation, and misdirection. Imagination both creates and counteracts these problems.

DELIBERATE PRACTICE

Still, using your imagination can help you more fully perceive what it's like in the doctor's shoes and the patient's shoes. As Dr. Thomas Gilovich says, there's "a direct link between imagination and perception". To imagine and perceive with accuracy, practice is necessary. True practice is what Dr. Anders Ericsson has dubbed, "deliberate practice". In deliberate practice, you don't just repeat the same thing the same way; instead, like the movie *Groundhog Day,* you should learn from your mistakes and do it differently the next time. In deliberate practice, a particular skill is focused on, with immediate feedback. With proper coaching or teaching, you are told what you are doing wrong, what you are doing correctly, and what you can do to improve. With such feedback and attention, you can make great strides; and the reverse is true as well – in the absence of appropriate

DELIBERATE PRACTICE: THE VIOLIN

When I was younger, practicing violin was the closest I got to deliberate practice. The goal each week wasn't to get better (although that did happen over time) but to practice one or two songs and be able to play them perfectly. I had a weekly private lesson, and my teacher, who I privately thought was a sweaty troll, would listen to each note I played and correct each and every one. He would sometimes mark certain passages that I should play repetitively, until I got them right. He would assign scales or discrete tasks (e.g. work on vibrato for five minutes a day). He would point out all my mistakes. Immediate feedback and learning from mistakes were part of my practice, through his teaching.

Rather than valuing his instruction, I hated it. I hated practicing the violin, and it was impossible to like a teacher who I boxed into the category of a fairy-tale monster. I disliked him with an unusual intensity. It's too bad; in retrospect, he was the best teacher of deliberate practice that I have had. As a child, however, I didn't comprehend the value of what he was teaching me. I didn't realize that the troll had magic.

feedback, you will probably struggle with forward progress. In deliberate practice, there must be a defined goal, with terms of reaching that goal.

The two important elements of deliberate practice are as follows: 1. A goal that ideally can be broken up into measurable, actionable tasks, and 2. Immediate feedback. Deliberate practice takes effort, and Dr. Ericsson suggests that you can do no more than two to four hours of deliberate practice in one consecutive time block, given the degree of focus and concentration that is required. You must have an internally generated desire and will for deliberate practice.

Once the resolve is there, you need to know what to practice. For sports and music, practice is more obvious – dribbling or kicking a ball, karate movements, swimming laps, playing scales on an instrument. Sports and music have clearly delineated associated skills that can be practiced, especially under the guidance of a dedicated coach or teacher. In many fields, it takes years to become an expert, as the process is not dependent on knowledge and skills alone but multifaceted decision-making that develops in a time-dependent fashion through experience and exposure.

Deliberate practice is challenging. But there is good news. In the Science of Well-Being, Yale University's most popular course of all-time, Dr. Laurie Santos quotes Mihaly Csikszentmihalyi: "The best moments in our lives are not the passive, receptive, relaxing times. The best moments usually occur if a person's body or mind is stretched to the limits in a voluntary effort to accomplish something difficult and worthwhile." Dr. Csikszentmihalyi is a Hungarian-American psychologist who published the book, *Flow*. He demonstrated that optimal flow happens when your strengths and skills are put to the test and you feel the right amount of difficulty. Challenge may be different for each individual. Challenge and deliberate practice go hand-in-hand. It may be counterintuitive, but ultimately the challenge will create pleasure.

Doctors already are experienced with deliberate practice, in medical and surgical practices, from medical school, through residency, and beyond. Patients come to see doctors because of their experience generated through the practice of medicine and surgery. Diagnostic and technical skills are essential and take time to learn and develop; training is long and arduous. Doctors practice and have practiced these skills continuously and carefully throughout their careers.

Patients, particularly those with chronic medical problems, can become very experienced with healthcare. Patients know how hard it may be to get an appointment, how long they may need to wait before being seen, how testing may be arduous and inconclusive. Patients who are familiar with the healthcare system in this way often learn to self-advocate, finding the doctors and healthcare staff that are able to best guide them, the appointments that work best in their schedules, the fastest way to get questions answered.

Meanwhile, it is also essential to practice toward optimal doctor-patient connection. Doctors and patients must not forget about seeing and showing their individual humanity to each other. Because "humanity" and "connection" can seem like abstract concepts without obvious, concrete steps to take to practice toward establishing them, discrete, "smarter" goals can help, focusing on what is perceived as two individuals interact.

SPORTS AND DELIBERATE PRACTICE

The goalie is Asian, like me, but with short hair trimmed close to her head. She is "off her line", way too far in front of the goal, when Carli Lloyd gets possession of the ball near the middle of the field. The next sequence is almost instantaneous, but I had time to hold my breath. A beat of a heart, and Carli Lloyd looks at the goalie and the goal behind her. The goalie sees this shift in gaze and frantically back-pedals toward the goal, predicting but unable to prevent what is to come. Another quick heartbeat and Carli Lloyd powerfully kicks the ball toward the goal, and it sails perfectly above the goalie's head, falling in sync with her body as she throws herself backward in an unsuccessful attempt to block the ball, which drops into the goal, her body onto turf. I exhale as the cheers erupt around me and on screen.

This stunning kick represents the third goal by the US Women's Team in just 16 minutes, and the US women go on to win the game and seal the 2015 World Cup title. Never dreaming that such an opportunity would present itself in game play, much less in a World Cup final, Carli Lloyd had deliberately practiced that very kick over years of training.

SMARTER GOALS

A useful mnemonic in setting up deliberate practice is SMARTER. Using the SMARTER mnemonic, you can gauge how to practice what you need, based on your particular situation. SMARTER can measure your efforts. SMARTER stands for **S**pecific, **M**easurable, **A**chievable, **R**elevant, **T**ime-bound, **E**valuated, and **R**eviewed. For a particular sport like tennis, instead of just saying, "I want to get better", deliberate practice would be practice aimed at a specific goal like developing a better serve. Relevant practice can be measured and achieved in a time-bound fashion by saying, "I want to be able to serve the tennis ball correctly 9 out of 10 times within a month's time." You can then evaluate and review in one month if your practice got you to your goal.

> "Isn't it a bit unnerving that doctors call what they do practice?"
> — George Carlin, American Stand-Up Comedian, Amateur Philosopher and Author

FEEDBACK

Once you create goals directed at practicing toward good medicine, critique of your practice is critical. I used to dread feedback, positive or negative.

Compliments embarrassed me, constructive criticism could level me, unfiltered comments could destroy my psyche for too long. My instinct was to summarily avoid all feedback – nothing good came of it. However, feedback is necessary to refine whatever you create and complete, including any efforts toward doctor-patient connection. Although I have not always set a good example of appreciating feedback, I became fully invested in feedback, particularly as I realized how much I learn from it. I came to value feedback more readily once I developed a "growth mindset", championed most popularly by Dr. Carol Dweck in her book *Mindset: The New Psychology of Success*. Hard work, challenge, failing – I appreciate these things more and more, and most of all it is comforting that failing is necessary. Failing is actually a good thing.

In a growth mindset, improvement happens with work; challenges are necessary for improvement. Hard work or effort comes before learning, and doing something should feel hard. Failing is useful because it shows you how to improve. Challenges that may result in failing are sought out. The fixed mindset is the opposite of this, and in that mindset, improvement is a result of innate talent and smarts, with anything challenging suggesting you are not good enough, that you are out of your league. Individuals with a fixed mindset want things to feel easy, failure is not an option, and challenges are avoided (see **Appendix**).

Connecting between doctors and patients becomes easier when you use a growth mindset to 1) create a sense of the patient (or doctor) as if you are in their shoes, 2) practice doing this because you will fail (I continue to do so, sometimes miserably), and 3) learn from your own critique of the process. Critique is dependent on subjective context, unique to you as an individual, dependent on your values, desires, and goals.

While most of us fail more than we succeed, confronting failure can be difficult. Others' failings and failures are often kept private, so any failing or failure you see in yourself can be devastating. Knowing that others fail helps counteract this detrimental feeling. A recent study emphasized that if students are taught that all people fail, including geniuses in the history books like Albert Einstein and Marie Curie, students perform better and work harder. The base knowledge that failure is a given creates a growth mindset.

Failure does not mean that one lacks the ability to accomplish something. Failing and learning from failure may need to be part of the process of reliably establishing doctor-patient connection (if it happens easily the first try, all the better). Failing sets up the goals you need to aim for. Ultimately, failure teaches you the most, shining a light on what can be worked on for continued forward progress. Dr. Rana Awdish, author of *In Shock: My Journey from Death to Recovery and the Redemptive Power of Hope* writes, "As a patient, I was privy to failures that I'd been blind to as a clinician. There were disturbing deficits in communication, uncoordinated care, and occasionally an apparently complete absence of empathy. I recognized myself in every failure." Dr. Awdish also suggests there is hope, as by "illuminating our failures, we can begin an authentic conversation about shared purpose, resilience, and building an engaged culture".

KEY TAKEAWAY

Ideally, the medical *and* psychosocial aspects of doctoring would be practiced, the latter through perceiving, imagining, and implementing optimal care and connection. To me, it is healthy healthcare relationships that encompass medical and social diagnosis – it is doctors fully appreciating a patient's humanity in order to give them necessary, realistic hope while giving the right diagnosis and treatment; it is patients being willing to nudge doctors, if and when possible, to remind them to do so. Perceiving a person (whether doctor or patient) accurately is dependent on metaperception (thinking about what is seen, heard, and felt); as you are not always going to be right, you have to be open to feedback. It may take time to establish good relationship-centered care through doctor-patient connection, it may not happen instantly on the first visit, and open communication between doctor and patient with necessary feedback is helpful.

Most doctors became doctors so that they could care for patients. Most patients did not intend to be patients. Healthcare is increasingly depersonalized due to time constraints, bureaucratic rules, and insurance issues. Metaperception can put focus back on what can truly make a difference in good medicine – the humanity of both patients and doctors.

IMAGINE OPTIMAL DOCTOR-PATIENT CONNECTION

Visual Perception:* For five minutes, picture good medicine in a healthcare interaction, either mentally or by watching a video (e.g. a healthcare interaction in a movie) and mimic that interaction for a minute, watching yourself in a mirror or videotaping yourself and watching the playback. After watching yourself, compare yourself to the relationship you are mimicking. What did you see and mimic?

Auditory Perception:* Set aside five minutes to think about what good medicine in a strong healthcare relationship sounds like. Mimic those qualities and words for a minute, recording yourself and listening to what you sound like. What did you hear and try to mimic?

Emotional Perception:* Mentally imagine for five minutes good medicine in a healthcare relationship you are in or saw on a screen. Write down the emotions that were expressed, either with body language, tone of voice, or words. Mimic those emotions by watching yourself in a mirror or recording yourself for one minute. When you watch yourself, write down the emotions you see and compare with the emotions you were trying to express. What is effective, and what is not? What did you feel and mimic?

*These perceptive modalities are covered in more

THE IMPORTANCE OF IMAGINATION: REALISTIC HOPE FOR THE FUTURE

It takes imagination to mentally trace a given outcome and allow alignment of your practice, expectations, and goals. In my son's case, when I learned that he was deaf I initially believed, as do many, that deafness precludes oral language fluency. I was wrong. While I wanted to optimize spoken language because I had the mental image in my head of my own daughter and other children babbling and speaking,* I had trouble believing that my son would achieve the same, partly because the doctors we saw confirmed my preconceived notion of deafness being synonymous with signed language, telling us that my son was unlikely to achieve spoken language. As my innate bias was reinforced by our healthcare team, hope for spoken language seemed unrealistic. Despite these predictions, realistic hope for spoken language grew slowly but surely as I saw my

> "Imagination is more important than knowledge. For knowledge is limited, whereas imagination embraces the entire world, stimulating progress, giving birth to evolution."
> — Albert Einstein, Theoretical Physicist

son's progress and met and heard other deaf children and parents of deaf children speaking of their past experiences navigating a similar journey.

I know I wasn't alone in my bias, because when my son was about four years old, we participated with 15 other international families in a three-week intensive language program at the John Tracy Clinic in Los Angeles. One of the other parents, a likable Irish woman with a ready smile and warm manner, had a four-year-old daughter with a unilateral cochlear implant. She shared with me that hearing my son's language ability (which at the time was still severely delayed) had made her appreciate what could be possible. In Ireland, where they lived, experts considered signed language the language of the deaf, and a diagnosis of deafness came with the bias that spoken language was impossible. Seeing my son and others in the American program, she was more able to imagine her own beautiful daughter achieving greater spoken language ability. Real-life experience gave her hope and a goal.

Even without seeing or hearing someone or something right in front of you, imagination can provide the means for realistic hope for the future.

Research has shown that creating a mental image activates many of the same areas in the brain as actually perceiving a real-life object. The same is true for perceiving a sound around you versus imagining that same sound. Imagining yourself feeling fear also can trigger the same pathways in the brain as the identical spontaneously generated emotion.

We all have limitations, but to a certain degree, those limitations are created by the boundaries we set for our abilities, many due to our implicit biases. Diverse mentors and role models are increasingly emphasized as real-life examples to help us overcome our prejudices and allow for greater and varied achievements. If ever an exact replica of what you desire is lacking (and truly, when is there ever such a replica, as each of us individually is unique), you can imagine, dream big, and forge something new. Throughout history, there are untold examples of this in the United States alone – Elizabeth Blackwell being the first woman doctor; Barack Obama being the first black president; Helen Keller being blind, deaf, and mute yet attending college, teaching, and writing.

---

*I have nothing against signed language; new parenthood is daunting enough without adding fluency in an entirely new language.

ACTING AS AN EMPATHY TOOL

When you see someone act, they are putting themselves in another person's shoes, creating an entirely new persona that may be completely different from his/her true personality, in order to evoke a particular character for those watching. Acting is a type of grand illusion, through which the best actors and actresses are able to portray someone else, using a harmonious combination of appearance, including clothing and makeup, body language, vocalization, and emotions. Acting is an art and a craft.

The beauty of acting is that it can break open entirely new experiences for the actor/actress and the viewer. Seeing a familiar actor/actress take on an entirely new role and make it believable is a demonstration of the fine balance between what is truly there (i.e. one's true character) and what is imagined and portrayed (i.e. the role being played). Doctors and patients both act a certain way in their interactions, not to say that either are putting on a show, pretending, or play-acting. But imagining what is optimal and practicing that in real time can make a positive difference toward genuine connections that are stronger. Great actors, through practicing their craft, can make a character authentic, believable, and convincing. While doctors and patients should not just be role-playing, particularly in serious medical situations, practicing toward relatable, strong, and open doctor-patient relationships is worthwhile. Indeed, two thespians that are much beloved by many, Meryl Streep and Robert De Niro, both believe that acting (taking on the role of another) can promote empathy toward others. Similarly, if a doctor practices, even just once or twice, taking on the role of a patient, and a patient also does the same for the role of doctor, both doctors and patients will likely have a better understanding of the other.

"You have to be able to put yourself in somebody else's shoes. Only then can you understand their emotions and reasons, even though you do not agree with them."
— Robert De Niro, American Actor

FURTHER READING

27 Remain "professional" and patients try to remain "composed", it is harder to sense the other's private world…Lelorain S, et al. How does a physician's accurate understanding of a cancer patient's unmet needs contribute to patient perception of physician empathy? *Patient Educ Couns* 2015;98:734-741. AND Campbell JA. Person centered theory and considerations for counseling, practice, and teaching. *Global Engagement and Transformation* 2018;2. AND Rogers CR. The necessary and sufficient conditions of therapeutic personality change. *J Consulting Psychol* 1957;21:95-103.

28 "the contours of their lives, at least once, from the inside."…Gavin F. An imaginative partnership: Parents and the doctors who care for their children. *Paediatr Child Health* 2009;14(5):295-297.

29 "…we listen not only with our ears"…Robertson K. Active listening: more than just paying attention. *Aust Fam Physician* 2005;34:1053-1055.

30 Seeing, hearing, and feeling during a health-care interaction to construct an image of a given patient…Gavin F. *Paedtr Child Health* 2009;14:295-297.

30 Dr. Maltz researched this phenomenon and suggested that our mental image of ourselves… Maltz M. *Psycho-cybernetics: A New Way to Get More Living Out of Life.* North Hollywood:

Wilshire Book Co, 1976.

32 Deliberate practice…Ericsson KA. Deliberate practice and acquisition of expert performance: A general overview. *Acad Emerg Med* 2008;15:988-994. AND Ericsson KA, Harwell KW. Deliberate practice and proposed limits on the effects of practice on the acquisition of expert performance: Why the original definition matters and recommendations for future research. *Front Psychol* 2019;10:2396.

37 Carli Lloyd…Lloyd C. *All Heart: My Dedication and Determination to Become One of Soccer's Best.* New York: Houghton Mifflin Harcourt, 2016.

38 SMARTER GOALS…Doran GT. There's a S.M.-A.R.T. way to write management's goals and objectives. *Management Review* 1981;70:35–36. AND Macleod L. Making SMART goals smarter. *Physician Executive* 2013;38:68-70. AND https://www.wanderlustworker.com/setting-s-m-a-r-t-e-r-goals-7-steps-to-achieving-any-goal/

39 Once I developed a "growth mindset"…Dweck C. *Mindset: The New Psychology of Success.* New York: Ballantine Books, 2008. AND Blackwell LS, Trzesniewski KH, Dweck CS. Implicit theories of intelligence predict achievement across an adolescent transition: A longitudinal study and an intervention. *Child Development* 2007; 78(1):246–263. AND Yeager DS, Miu AS, Powers J, Dweck CS. Implicit theories of personality and attributions of hostile intent: A meta-analysis, an experiment, and a longitudinal intervention. *Child Development* 2013;84(5):1651-1667.

40 A recent study emphasized that if students are taught that all people fail...Lin-Siegler X, Ahn JN. Even Einstein struggled: Effects of learning about great scientists' struggles on high school students' motivation to learn science. *J Educ Psychol* 2016;108(3):314-328.

41 Dr. Rana Awdish...Awdish RLA. A View from the Edge — Creating a Culture of Caring. *New England Journal of Medicine* 2017;376(1):7-9.

"...shared purpose, resilience, and building an engaged culture."...Ibid.

46 Actually perceiving a real-life object...Boccia M, Sulpizio V, Teghil A, et al. The dynamic contribution of the high-level visual cortex to imagery and perception. *Human Brain Mapping* 2019;40(8):2449-2463. AND Dijkstra N, Bosch SE, Van Gerven MAJ. Shared Neural Mechanisms of Visual Perception and Imagery. *Trends in Cognitive Sciences* 2019;23(5):423-434.

46 Imagining that same sound...Halpern AR, Zatorre RJ, Bouffard M, Johnson JA. Behavioral and neural correlates of perceived and imagined musical timbre. *Neuropsychologia* 2004;42(9):1281-1292.

46 Spontaneously generated emotion...Reddan MC, Wager TD, Schiller D. Attenuating Neural Threat Expression with Imagination. *Neuron* 2018;100(4):994-1005.e1004.

2 METACOGNITION: THINKING ABOUT WHAT YOU DO IN HEALTHCARE INTERACTIONS

"To think you know when you do not is a disease. Recognizing this disease as a disease is to be free of it."
— Lao Tzu, Chinese Philosopher

As a dermatology resident, I am standing outside the clinic room, presenting the patient's history of present illness and my findings on physical examination to my attending, the experienced dermatologist who is teaching me that day. I tell her that the patient is a middle-aged woman who has had bumps (the proper dermatologic term being "papules") on the anterior neck, the outsides of her arms and the front of her legs for a couple of months. The bumps are asymptomatic and are the tiniest bit shiny but kind of blend into her skin. She has no significant past medical history. My attending asks me what the patient has, and I tell her that I am not sure. She smiles at me, and without having yet seen the patient, she tells me that the patient has eruptive syringomas. Her initial impression outside the room does not change once she enters, and later, when I look up eruptive syringomas in a textbook, the images look exactly like the skin of the patient in clinic. I am inordinately impressed by my attending, and she shrugs it off – this is dermatology, she says. With the right description, you can imagine what the patient looks like, and seeing it in your mind, you can know what the patient has. Notice also that this example demonstrates how diagnosis can be a largely cerebral activity, and the patient wasn't even present!

The same thing happened innumerable times as I sat at the microscope with my first mentor in dermatopathology, Dr. Ronald Barr. In my initial months staring down at pink and blue tissue sections gloriously magnified by the microscope, I had absolutely no idea what I was looking at. Dr. Barr would render diagnoses for different things, and I simply could not see what he was seeing. I knew he wasn't making things up – he had the ability to see things that I could not. Using his vast treasure trove of memory, he would say that a certain slide looked like an entity that was described in a journal article, "Oh, maybe about 3 years ago." And someone sitting at the microscope with him, sometimes me, sometimes someone else, would go to one of the neatly organized piles of journals, stacked together and wrapped in bundles by rubber bands, to find the right article. It wasn't quite like an online search, but somehow better, the mystery of how he could translate what a slide looked like, link it to his memory of something he had read even years before, and then direct us to a particular pile on the floor of his office – "Check that stack right there." It was amazing. He was rather blasé about his abilities, telling me, "Christine, once you've been doing this for as long as I have, things have to kind of stick."

The same type of rapid-fire generation of medical diagnosis happens in other specialties, not just dermatology and dermatopathology. The COVID-19 pandemic affected us worldwide in the spring of 2020, and many of my colleagues and I volunteered to serve on the medical wards during the acute period of surging infections in the United States, to help alleviate the extreme time commitment that was falling on internal medicine physicians in particular. In the short time I volunteered, I had all-important backup by seasoned, inpatient medical attendings and also had two experienced residents, one of whom was graduating in one month from her program and was for all intents and purposes an attending herself. Because I was so far from medical school and my intern year, I did do a crash course in medicine online, relearning the newest algorithms and management of heart failure, acute kidney injury, inpatient diabetes mellitus, and other topics. I wrote notes in a small notebook that was my constant companion while I attended on the wards. And for me, one of the best things about volunteering actually was, somewhat tellingly, not directly patient-related. The experience brought back nostalgia for my intern year, how I learned medicine in real time, through residents senior to me and more experienced than me; guiding me, teaching me, asking me questions on what I thought the patient had, what I wanted to do as the next step, what else I needed to check given a certain symptom or a certain laboratory test. I saw the soon-to-graduate resident in action, discussing cases with me and the first-year resident-in-training (who knew more internal medicine than I did!), rapidly checking laboratory values, examining radiologic findings herself through uploaded material in the medical record, weighing probabilities of what each patient had, what we could do for them, when they might be able to go home. I was reminded in real time of how you learn through seeing, doing, teaching – the cases that we see teach us, then we see the same case again and do what worked the last time, and then teach others what we have learned. There are algorithms and protocols, and there were specific ones for COVID-19. In the midst of this, I remembered the mantra I had learned so long ago in medical school, no scarier now than then – *See one, do one, teach one.* A mantra I still believe in, but one that potentially reduces patients to a medical diagnosis or procedure.

There is a feeling of power and control in doctoring, and the transition into being on the "other side" of healthcare can be very jarring for doctors, particularly for potentially life-altering diagnoses. When I first thought that my son was deaf, healthcare data, in this case auditory sound booth testing, contradicted my instinct. The doctor told me that my son was fine, but we could return for a follow-up test since he was just nine months old. At 13 months of age, the auditory sound booth testing again was interpreted by the doctor as normal. The doctor's assessment and the test data were against my own gut feeling derived from being around my son on a daily basis. When we finally got the right diagnosis of auditory neuropathy and *objective* evidence of my son's fluctuating hearing that was, at its worst, profound deafness (no sound at all), it pained me for a long time that I had not trusted myself.

This experience ultimately helped shape me, and from then on, I refused to let medical data override the personal data that we had from living our own stories on a day-to-day basis. I forced myself to ask when things didn't match up; I made myself try to not take it too personally if doctors seemed reluctant to answer (or would refuse to answer). I would just ask again, or ask someone else, or ask for a second opinion, until the answers made sense in light of our own daily experience. It was not about getting the answer that I wanted but best answers for our experience in light of the best expertise of our medical professionals.

DOCTORS AND DIAGNOSIS

If you are a doctor or healthcare professional, there are certain things that you already do for patient care. (If you are not a doctor or a healthcare professional and you are a patient, read this to learn how your doctors think, or skip on to the next section.) As a doctor, these are some of the things you[1] do – you can read about a patient case or hear someone talk about a case and accurately make the diagnosis; you can take one abnormal laboratory test or one patient symptom and navigate through a patient's chart or history, fitting the puzzle pieces together into a coherent whole; in seconds, you can paint a mental picture of what a patient looks like, their skin or their physical examination, determine what

---

[1] In this section, "you", "your", and "yourself" refers to doctors.

is most probable for a diagnosis, and when you see that patient, your mental picture can sometimes be exactly correct depending on how good the initial description was; you can listen to yourself or others create a list of possibilities for a patient's diagnosis and rank the possibilities in terms of probability and ways to further evaluate and eliminate those choices to land on one diagnosis; you know that diagnosis is fluid, that you are not always right, that you can be wrong, that you can do better. You also know that while doctoring can be a calling and not just a way to pass eight-plus hours of the day, it can be trying and exhausting and Sisyphean because patient problems do not disappear because it is 5 pm. You know that the energy and excitement you had at first receiving your medical degree and seeing patients on your own for the first time dissipates, that the days can be long and at the same time too short, that not every patient survives. You know that some patients are sicker than others, that some diagnoses (like cancer) are scarier than others, that your training is not always sufficient to guide you toward the perfect next step. Sometimes you make things up as you go along or you try it because it seems like the best choice or the only alternative. You cannot help, over time, to become desensitized to some degree because it is the normal course of things that as novelty wears off, things become routine. And yet you know, to a greater or lesser degree depending on your own emotional state each day, that what is routine to you is often novel to your patient. And the best doctors know that what is novel to the patient should be treated as unique by the doctor.

Doctors and healthcare professionals spend a lot of time on diagnosis and treatment, because these things are critical to patient care. In my fields of dermatology and dermatopathology, both visual specialties in which diagnosis is largely based on visual recognition, visual perception is important to diagnosis. In medicine in general, visual perception is used to assess a patient's general appearance (e.g. very sick vs. healthy-appearing) and visual portions of the physical examination. What is seen is evaluated, carefully and methodically. Mentally imagining a patient's insides and the potential organs involved (termed a mental CT scan as you are visualizing "slices" of the body much as a radiologic study would) improves the generation of potential diagnoses for a patient. What is heard is also weighed systematically. History taking is carefully taught to medical students. Doctors are trained in this and know how to ask the right medical questions and parse the correct medical data on an almost automatic basis; in addition to words, doctors are also trained to listen to the heart, lungs, and digestive tract.

But there is also a psychosocial aspect of patient care, and this was never overtly taught to me, although it was the reason that I wanted to become a doctor. I imagined myself caring for patients, making a difference in their lives, helping them. In reality, I believe a lot of doctors burn out because daily schedules can feel like an inefficient grind, the things accomplished (or not) wrapped in bureaucracy, and it doesn't necessarily always seem like doctors make a difference for patients. But it doesn't have to be this way. Burnout has less chance of taking hold when doctors and patients connect over the right medical diagnosis while incorporating the psychosocial aspects of care.

PATIENTS AND HEALTHCARE

Even if you do not work in the healthcare field, it is the

rare person that is never once a patient. As a patient or the family member of a patient, there are certain things that you[2] already do when you encounter healthcare. These are some of the things you do – you may trust the information given by your doctor and leave it at that. You may go a bit (or a lot) further. You may consult with friends or family with or without healthcare experience. You can read about what your doctor told you or listen to what your doctor and others have to say about a particular diagnosis; you may take your abnormal laboratory tests or studies or your symptom(s) and surf the internet, fitting the puzzle pieces together as you can; you may compare what you have and were told you have to descriptions that you find as you look things up; you may read about other possibilities for your diagnosis and rank the possibilities in terms of probability and ways to further evaluate and eliminate those choices to land on one diagnosis. Sometimes you may think your doctor is not right, but in general, you are too polite to say so. Most times, you may not doubt that the doctor is right; you know that there were years of training involved to do what your doctor does.

---

[2]In this section, "you", "your", and "yourself" refers to patients or patient family members.

But sometimes you may not actually trust the doctor you saw, and you experience firsthand that by seeing another doctor, you get another diagnosis! Doctors don't always agree, in which case, one of them must be wrong. You know that sometimes it seems like your doctor doesn't have enough time for you, or the doctor doesn't call you back as quickly as you would want. You know how busy your doctor probably is, but sometimes you really need that doctor to pay attention to you, and it might be at an inconvenient time. You know that the doctor may not be able to solve everything, but you need someone there that should know about your healthcare problems in exacting detail. You want to know that if you are really sick, or have a scary diagnosis, that your doctor will know precisely what to do and how to fix things. With all that, as a bonus, you may like your doctor, and as in any important relationship, it is nice if the doctor likes you back. And you know, to a greater or lesser degree depending on your own emotional state each day, that what is routine to the doctor is often new to you as a patient; the medical terms that roll easily off the doctor's tongue are often a nonsensical foreign language. And because of all this, you have a sense that the best doctor will hold your hand through it all, but unless you've experienced that, it's hard to know what it would feel like.

METACOGNITION

Using terms from behavioral economics, thinking about the way doctors and patients think is metacognition, and there is both fast and slow thinking, termed System 1 and System 2 thinking by Dr. Daniel Kahneman. The rapid processing used when a doctor knows in seconds what a patient has is System 1 thinking – it is essentially pattern recognition. Everyone does this, not just doctors – pattern recognition is how you recognize faces, animals, houses, cars, logos, and even book covers. In contrast to the instant recognition example of System 1 (fast thinking), System 2 takes time. This slower process is no less valuable, and System 2 can be used to check the quick decisions that System 1 makes. The reverse is true as well – System 1 can be used to check conclusions that System 2 makes. Both Systems are valuable, and both can lead to error.

Consider the following:

1+1 = ?
What is the answer, spelled out, of one added to one?

Because 1 + 1 is familiar to you, it is "easy", and you can very quickly come to the correct answer of 2. With the second question, it is much less familiar to add numbers when they are spelled out, and it is even less common to be asked to spell the answer out as "t-w-o". For tasks outside the norm, even though the answer remains easy, slower, System 2 thinking takes over. Taking more time does not mean that you don't know the answer. And taking less time doesn't mean that your answer is worse.

For me, a total body skin examination is now "easy". I have been training for years – it is like 1 +1 = 2. I can examine someone "quickly" – many patients tell me they are surprised that I have finished examining them – but the rapid processing that I can use for a skin examination doesn't mean that I am being sloppy. I can even "pretend" to go slower with my examination, but just as 1+1 = 2 no matter how slowly I try to calculate it, a slower skin examination doesn't necessarily mean more accurate. What I have found does help me is to deliberately observe the skin from different angles, from when I first encounter the patient and they are sitting in a chair next to the examination table – the light hits their skin in a different way than when they move to the examination table. I can look at them again as they sit on the examination table, and again from a different angle as they lie down, flip over, flip over again. I can walk around the patient, because that also changes my perspective just a little, and I see things a different way. I also appreciate it when patients tell me from the outset if they are concerned about anything in particular, as I can focus deliberately on that as well, using both System 1 and 2 processing. Because I have done skin exams countless times, I have a routine, and it is largely System 1 that directs me to do what I do in a skin examination, with System 2 jumping in at the proper times.

Most people, including me, like System 1 thinking because it is easy and comfortable. But System 1 makes mistakes – System 1 is at the root of implicit biases, prejudices, and stereotypes. System 2 creates error, too, and ideally both systems are used in a balanced fashion as in my detailed skin examinations.

You cannot question every decision that you make; it is an impossible task. As Dr. Kahneman writes, "System 2 is much too slow and inefficient to serve as a substitute for System 1 in making routine decisions. The best we can do is a compromise: learn to recognize situations in which mistakes are likely and try harder to avoid significant mistakes when the stakes are high."

In important healthcare interactions, the stakes can be very high.

Try to calculate this quickly, without thinking too hard.

> ## If whitewater rafting costs $110, and this includes a set of photos from the trip, how much is the rafting alone if the rafting is $100 more than the cost of the photos?

This problem is adapted from one of Dr. Kahneman's in *Thinking: Fast and Slow*. The quick, System 1 answer for most people, including me, is that the rafting costs $100, and the photos cost $10. However, this is incorrect because while $100 more than $10 is $110, rafting ($110) plus photos ($10) would be $120 rather than a total of $110. The rafting must be $105 and the photos $5, in order for the rafting to be $100 more than photos alone if the total is $110 altogether. I will admit that I tend to get this type of question wrong over and over again. (Even though my intuitive, gut answer is wrong, I don't consider myself to be bad at math!)

System 1 is useful because it creates ease. System 1 is the source of your biases, but also your efficiencies, your ability to think as an expert. When doctors come to an instant diagnosis, System 1 is at play. But System 1 can be wrong, unfortunately, and doctors can be wrong – an immediate, fast diagnosis might not be right. For something high stakes like a critical medical diagnosis, it is important to check intuition with reflective, careful System 2 reasoning.

You may think, then, that System 2 is better than System 1. But System 2 makes mistakes as well. How can System 2 lead you astray? A good analogy is not seeing the forest for the trees. Focusing on details that are not necessarily relevant to a diagnosis (while of course not realizing this to be the case) can make you lose sight of the bigger picture. I can see System 2 errors as I teach students and residents dermatology and dermatopathology, teaching them to perceive what a skin finding or a microscopic finding can tell them. Students and residents know a lot – they are all very smart – but there is always at least one instance when they unintentionally, inappropriately focus on something that leads them away from the correct diagnosis, and this is true for me as well (although much harder and sometimes impossible for me to see myself doing it in the moment).

In my own practice, I have realized that medical diagnosis is optimally based on *both* System 1 and System 2. If System 1 provides an immediate diagnosis, I should still check it (and this can be done fairly quickly) with System 2. If System 1 does not give me a diagnosis, I can use System 2 to try to figure something out. These patterns of thinking are complementary, and the more I use System 2, more of what I see becomes integrated into System 1, freeing up my thinking processes to observe even more.

CLINICAL EMPATHY

While observation and listening as components of coming to a medical diagnosis are essential to doctoring, doctor-patient connection is best established through clinical empathy, which can be considered "the backbone of the patient-physician relationship". The same thinking tools used in listening to a medical history and observing in a patient examination can be applied to create more comprehensive patient care that integrates the correct medical diagnosis with clinical empathy. Empathy decreases burnout. What is felt by the patient, as perceived and understood by the doctor – this is empathy. More specifically, *cognitive* empathy in medicine can be defined as *understanding* what a patient feels (not necessarily feeling it yourself) and being able to communicate your understanding with an intention to help. *Affective* empathy is relatively automatic and can be likened to sympathy or the feeling of compassion. *Clinical* empathy enmeshes both cognitive and affective empathy as specifically applied to the patient-doctor interaction. While there are many other definitions of empathy, clinical empathy, and particularly cognitive empathy, is a skill.

Considering clinical empathy, you may think, as I did for many years, that medical diagnosis and treatment plans are what doctors should focus on. And this is indeed what I did, with studies supporting that increasing experience in the healthcare field can erode empathy, as it did for me. Medical students, physicians, and nurses early on in training are more empathetic than later on in their careers. That was true for me, someone who started out wanting to make a difference for people but got turned around by how overwhelming learning medicine can be, how arduous the training can sometimes be, how distressing personal events can make doctoring other people's medical problems, at times, feel horribly burdensome.

I learned firsthand the importance of clinical empathy when I experienced it myself as the mother of a patient. Feeling seen by my mentor and my son's surgeon (see **Introduction**) was unexpected and inexplicably comforting. Their support did not supplant my son's medical diagnosis or my worry, but it gave me strength. To me, it was a sign of greatness, and I do believe all doctors aspire to be great.

While clinical empathy alone does not give patients the best healthcare experience, striking the right balance between clinical empathy and a focus on medical facts can happen with metacognitive attention. People overestimate their ability to accurately recognize emotions expressed in others' faces, and stress reduces empathy between strangers. Medical errors themselves increase healthcare worker stress, creating a vicious cycle of medical error generating stress, leading to decreased empathy and increased burnout, and further medical error. While the exact reasons why empathy declines with greater experience and training are unclear, it has been suggested that it could partially be due to a lack of empathic role models – students and residents are learning the patterns of behavior that they see in their teachers. It may also be due to habitually focusing on disease rather than the patient as a person.

As a medical student, I talked with my peers and teachers on innumerable occasions about proper history taking, diagnosis, and treatment. As a medical student, we sometimes did address the psychosocial aspects of what we were doing and would do. For example, as a first-year medical student, I learned anatomy on real cadavers, the smell of formaldehyde sticking to me, branding me a novitiate. We were exhorted by our teachers to uphold the dignity of each human being that had volunteered to further medical education with the gift of the bodies that we dissected and explored each day. The end of the course was marked by a candlelight ceremony during which our anonymous submissions regarding the process were read aloud, exploring our feelings and reactions to touching the body of another human being in such an abnormal, intimate fashion. I remember this experience as feeling sacred, although not all of my classmates felt the same way, and that was probably the last time we collectively spent time reflecting on what it felt like to do what we do, particularly when it is completely outside of normal, daily experience.

In contrast to the ceremony that accompanied my anatomy experience, the first patient of mine that died while under my care passed away inexplicably over a weekend. He had been admitted to the inpatient dermatology service for psoriasis, a common skin disorder that is not a cause of sudden death. Because it happened over the weekend, it was even harder to process what had taken place (I wasn't physically present at the time of death), and all I could find out was that he had had trouble breathing, was transferred from dermatology to medicine and then to the intensive care unit, where he died. There was never anyone to speak to about how I felt.

The silence surrounding that emotional event and subsequent ones suggested to me that to be strong, I should just move on. Ultimately, that is unhealthy, for both me and future patients. Allowing significant events, personal or work-related, to pass virtually unnoticed is unnatural and inhuman. Empathy for yourself and others is necessary.

USING METACOGNITION TOWARD CLINICAL EMPATHY

Empathy training does work, and such training is often through simulated patient encounters (see **Chapter 1,** Acting as an Empathy Tool, p. 47), with feedback on the trainee's performance. Medical students and some seasoned doctors may take such courses, but the vast majority of practicing doctors currently do not. Clinical empathy can be increased even without taking a formal course. On the simplest level, using metacognition to become more self-aware increases clinical empathy. For psychologists in training, mindfulness-based cognitive therapy is effective in increasing understanding of their own and patients' thoughts, feelings, behaviors, and bodily sensations. Although mindfulness-based cognitive therapy takes time to learn and use, its basic tenets include metacognitive awareness of thoughts and feelings in order to regulate emotional processing from automatic to conscious. For medical students, self-reflection, positive role models, and self-awareness promote the preservation and development of empathy. For undergraduate students, various interventions that foster self-awareness and reflection (including art, writing, drama, communication skills training, and simulated patient interviews) all increase empathy. While more research can be done, these studies support that empathy can be increased – it is a learnable skill through attention and awareness. Empathy is not just intuitive or emotional; it can be deliberate. Clinical empathy (and lack of such empathy) can be a learned response.

KEY TAKEAWAY

Optimizing doctor-patient connection for relationship-centered care can be achieved through metacognition, focusing not only on diagnosis and illness but also the doctor-patient interaction. You need to be aware, be able to recognize choices and potential actions, and be available to connect with yourself and others. While diagnosing and treating illness properly, doctors can take note of emotions, take the perspective of the patient while differentiating the patient from themselves, and gain understanding of the patient. Patients can also take note of emotions, become conscious of pressing needs and questions, and bring these to the doctor's attention. You can do all of this by using System 1 and 2 processing, which is already ingrained in the way you think. In the following chapters, I will talk about a few of my own healthcare experiences and expand on what you can do to reliably generate and maintain doctor-patient connection through using visual, auditory, and emotional habits. Through doing this, doctor-patient connection and relationship-centered care will grow stronger.

PRACTICAL APPLICATIONS

Consider how easy it is for you to drive home from somewhere familiar (System 1 thinking, fast thinking, instinctual). Compare this to driving somewhere new (System 2 thinking, slow thinking, analytical).

Think about your recent healthcare interactions. What were they like? What went well? What didn't go well?

METAPERCEPTION TOWARD CONNECTING WITH OTHERS

Visual Perception

What do you observe when you talk to someone else?
How important is body language?
How important is facial expression?
Do you prefer talking to someone in person or on the phone?

Auditory Perception

How well do you listen to others?
Does your mind wander?
How does tone of voice influence you?

Emotion Perception

What emotions do you tend to recognize in others?
How do you do this?
Through the words they are saying, facial expressions, body language, and/or tone of voice?

FURTHER READING

59 DOCTORS AND DIAGNOSIS...Elstein AS. Thinking about diagnostic thinking: A 30-year perspective. *Adv in Health Sci Educ* 2009;14:7-18.

61 Mentally imagining a patient's insides and the potential organs involved (termed a mental CT...Leeds FS et al. Teaching heuristics and mnemonics to improve generation of differential diagnosis. *Med Educ Online* 2020;25:1742967.

65 Using terms from behavioral economics... Kahneman D. *Thinking, Fast and Slow*. New York: Farrar, Straus and Giroux, 2011.

71 "the backbone of the patient-physician relationship."...Derksen F, et al. Effectiveness of empathy in general practice: A systematic review. *Br J Gen Pract* 2013;63:e76-84.

71 Empathy decreases burnout...Many articles; selected: Kim K. To feel or not to feel: Empathy and physician burnout. *Acad Psych* 2018;42:157-158. AND Silver J, et al. Mindfulness among genetic counselors is associated with increased empathy and work engagement and decreased burnout and compassion fatigue. *J Genet Couns* 2018;27:1175-1186. AND Salvarani V, et al. Protecting emergency room nurses from burnout: The role of dispositional mindfulness, emotion regulation and empathy. *J Nurs Manag* 2019;27:765-774. AND Samra R. Empathy and burnout in medicine – Acknowledging risks and opportunities. *J Gen Intern Med* 2018;33:991-993.

71   Empathy in medicine can be defined as understanding what a patient feels…Shamay-Tsoory S, et al. Two systems for empathy: a double dissociation between emotional and cognitive empathy in inferior frontal gyrus versus ventromedial prefrontal lesions. *Brain* 2009;132:617-627.

72   Experience in the healthcare field can erode empathy…Hojat M, et al. The devil is in the third year: A longitudinal study of erosion of empathy in medical school. *Acad Med* 2009;84:1182-1191. AND Han JL, et al. A review of empathy, its importance, and its teaching in surgical training. *J Surg Educ* 2018;75:88-94. AND Neumann M, et al. Empathy decline and its reasons: A systematic review of studies with medical students and residents. *Acad Med* 2011;86:996-1009.

72   Striking the right balance between clinical empathy and a focus on medical facts…https://www.scientificamerican.com/article/doctors-and-dehumanization-effect/

73   People overestimate their ability to accurately recognize emotions expressed in others' faces… Kelly KJ, et al. Metacognition of emotional face recognition. *Emotion* 2011;11:896-906.

73   And stress reduces empathy between strangers…Loren J et al. Reducing social stress elicits emotional contagion of pain in mouse and human strangers. *Curr Biol* 2015;doi:10.1016/j.cub.2014.11.028.

73   And further medical error…West CP, et al. Asso-

ciation of perceived medical errors with resident distress and empathy. *JAMA* 2006;296:1071-1078.

73 Due to a lack of empathic role models... Weissman S. Faculty empathy and the hidden curriculum. *Acad Med* 2012;87:389. AND Reisman AB. Outing the hidden curriculum. *Hastings Cent Rep* 2006;36:9. AND Wear D, et al. Can compassion be taught? Let's ask our students. *J Gen Intern Med* 2008;23:948-953.

75 Empathy training does work...Wundrich M, et al. Empathy training in medical students – a randomized controlled trial. *Med Teach* 2017;39:1096-1098.

76 Effective in increasing understanding of their own and patients' thoughts, feelings, behaviors, and bodily sensations...Rimes KA, et al. Pilot study of mindfulness-based cognitive therapy for trainee clinical psychologists. *Behav Cogn Psychother* 2011;39:235-241.

76 Metacognitive awareness of thoughts and feelings in order to regulate emotional processing from automatic to conscious... Herbert JD, et al. *Acceptance and Mindfulness in Cognitive Behavior Therapy: Understanding and Applying New Theories.* Hoboken: John Wiley & Sons, 2011.

76 Self-reflection, positive role models, and self-awareness promote the preservation and development of empathy...Seeberger A, et al. Can empathy be preserved in medical education? *Int J Med Educ* 2020;11:83-89.

76 All increase empathy...Batt-Rawden S, et al. Teaching empathy to medical students: an updated systematic review. *Acad Med* 2013;88:1171-1177.

76 Empathy is not just intuitive...Svedholm-Hakkinen A, et al. Intuitive and deliberative empathizers and systemizers. *J Pers* 2017;85:593-602. AND Heyes C. Empathy is not in our genes. *Neurosci Biobehav Rev* 2018;95:499-507.

77 Available to connect with yourself and others... Todaro-Franceschi V. The ART of maintaining the "care" in healthcare. *Nurs Manage* 2015;46:53-55.

77 Gain understanding of the patient...Jeffrey D. Empathy, sympathy and compassion in healthcare: Is there a problem? Is there a difference? Does it matter? *J R Soc Med* 2016;109:446-452.

3 DIAGNOSIS AND COGNITIVE BIAS: HOW YOUR THINKING CAN LEAD TO ERROR IN HEALTHCARE INTERACTIONS

"Nothing can harm you as much as your own thoughts unguarded."
— Buddha, Indian Philosopher and Religious Leader

The patient is a 50-year-old unemployed man who is unkempt. His hair looks unwashed, and he spontaneously apologizes that he smells bad; he tells me that he has not been able to shower for a couple of days due to problems with his water. He smells mildly of alcohol. His chief complaint is intense itchiness in his groin area, but also all over his body, for over six months. He tells me that he has seen many other doctors already, and no one has been able to find anything wrong with his skin. He lives with his 16-year-old daughter, and due to financial constraints, they sleep in the same bed. His daughter has no symptoms of itch and is healthy. He denies alcohol or drug use, has no other known medical problems, and his recent laboratory tests have been normal.

As I take this history, I note his disheveled appearance and the smell of liquor on his breath in spite of his denial of alcohol use. Itchiness has an extensive differential diagnosis, but common causes include dry skin in older adults and eczema/atopy in children. Internal disease of the liver or kidneys can cause itchiness, but he is reportedly healthy. While interviewing him, I look at the skin of his face, upper chest, and arms, and I do not see any specific findings. There are also no visible clues that he is itchy. There are no scratches to be seen.

I am tired, and I doubt that I will be able to give him a medical diagnosis given that multiple others have failed. Skin examination is standard in dermatology, and although I think that I won't find anything, I tell him I will briefly leave so he can undress completely and put a patient gown on. I want to examine the groin area since he told me his itching is the worst in that area. I feel reluctance to do this, maybe due to his appearance but also due to an inherent reticence, and I am momentarily grateful that he is the last patient of my morning.

I knock before entering to examine him. As is my custom, I start with his scalp and face and work downward as I examine his skin. He has back problems and does not want to lie down on the examination table, so he is standing as I examine the groin area.

I almost recoil when I see a minuscule crab-like bug adeptly and rapidly moving along the hairs of his lower abdomen. In an instant, the cause of his itchiness is apparent. Diagnosis: Pubic lice.

I think the diagnosis might be unwelcome news, but the patient bowls me over with his gratitude. He thanks me for looking, for giving him a diagnosis, for validating his concerns. He tells me that I am the first one of all the doctors he has seen to actually have examined him. (I feel guilty and disingenuous, but I don't confess to the lack of enthusiasm I had felt.) I tell him that it is my job to examine the skin, and he made the right decision to keep pursuing the cause of his itchiness by seeing a skin doctor. He tells me that he has seen other skin doctors, and I am the only one that believed him enough to examine him.

While I made the correct medical diagnosis and the patient was easily cured of the crab lice and the itchiness, I very well could have failed him. His appreciation made me feel more ashamed of myself. I only examined him because it is my standard practice – it is routine for me. Given his age, appearance, the smell of alcohol despite his denial of alcohol use, the inability of multiple previous doctors to give him a diagnosis (suggesting a high probability that he would have nothing on examination, as I hadn't known that no one had examined him), and the fact that his daughter was unaffected (suggesting against a parasite), I had favored (before the examination) that his itchiness was psychosomatic. I thought I had evidence supporting a high pretest probability that there would be nothing on examination. Diagnosis: Bias.

METACOGNITION IN DIAGNOSIS

This patient story illustrates several important concepts in thinking about proper diagnosis. During the patient interview and examination, I was using System 1 and 2 thinking (see **Chapter 2**). Dr. Daniel Kahneman, a Nobel-prize winning psychologist who pioneered the field of behavior economics, uses System 1 and System 2 as semantic markers of two major ways that you think. System 1 thinking is fast thinking, gut reactions. System 2 thinking is slow thinking, logical and analytical.

In the patient story above, System 1 (fast thinking) painted a picture for me of a patient with psychosomatic itch – denial of alcohol use while he smelled of it, absence of a working medical diagnosis after having seen multiple doctors. System 2 (slow thinking) seemed to be confirming my System 1 impression, as I mentally ran through common causes of itchiness without any seeming immediately likely. And while System 1 was leading me astray in terms of my favored diagnosis prior to the physical examination, it is also System 1 that allowed me to immediately recognize what was crawling on the patient.

Importantly, my standard practice of skin examination prevented my fatigue and my bias from obstructing the patient's care. Awareness of bias is important, but habitual, standard practice is also helpful to overcome bias in order to render optimal medical diagnosis and care.

BIAS IS COGNITIVE AND INTEGRAL TO HOW YOU THINK

Bias is integral to cognition and is generally a result of mental shortcuts ("rules of thumb" or "heuristics", another term coined by Dr. Daniel Kahneman, author of *Thinking, Fast and Slow*). These shortcuts are not necessarily bad (see **Appendix** for examples of cognitive bias). Your brain craves efficiency and will use any "rule of thumb" to help sift through the data that you are bombarded with at any given moment. One person's heuristic may be different from someone else's, and your cognitive biases are influenced by many things including your culture, education, goals, past experiences, outlook, and beliefs. Individual bias is why diverse opinions, and being aware of differences, helps decision-making and rendering a diagnosis.

Consider the following:

12

A 13 C

14

Interpretation can be based on past experience or context. In the first box, is the middle character a number or a letter? Read from left to right, I perceive it as a letter, "B". Read from top to bottom, I perceive it as a number, "13". Looking at data from different angles can lead to a different conclusion, and some may perceive the information in these boxes differently than I do.

12

13

14

A 13 C

HOW COGNITIVE BIAS APPLIES TO THE DOCTOR

Diagnosis is part of a physician's craft, both a process and a classification scheme. In terms of the latter, diagnosis rests on a pre-existing definition of what a given medical condition is. In terms of diagnosis as a process, patients do not come with labels that tell physicians what their set of symptoms and lab results mean. Physicians need to observe, listen, and think about how everything might tie together; this process leads to the medical diagnosis. The correct diagnosis aids positive health outcomes as subsequent decision-making rests on an accurate diagnosis. "Diagnosis remains fundamentally dependent on a personal interaction of a [clinician] with a patient, the sufficiency of communication between them, the accuracy of the patient's history and physical examination, and the cognitive energy necessary to synthesize a vast array of information."

Important considerations that overlay this diagnostic process include diagnostic uncertainty (doctors are often not 100% certain – a diagnosis is a hypothesis that needs to be supported by data), time (diseases evolve and can present in different ways over time), and population trends, including diversity. All of this involves clinical reasoning, which uses instinctive and analytical thinking patterns. Instinctive thinking involves pattern recognition as well as bias (bias is not inherently bad)– you've "seen" it before. But you often ignore, without even realizing, what you haven't "seen". Analytical thinking can help you see more, sometimes through checklists, standard practices and guidelines, and comparing conclusions from instinctive and analytical thinking.

Diagnosis is complex, and one study estimated that a physician would need to read about 29 hours/ workday to stay current with medical literature. As no one has this much time, proposed avenues for optimal diagnosis as knowledge continues to expand are team-based care, clinical practice guidelines, appropriate use criteria, and checklists. Diagnosis and avoidance of inappropriate bias are aided by getting help, from other doctors but also from patients.

Bias is often implicit, or hidden, until we consciously look for it. Particularly in healthcare, patients deserve to be looked at impartially, receiving the same level of care without damaging bias. While studies have shown that doctors are just as biased as the rest of the human population, this does not have to adversely affect clinical decision-making. Everyone has bias, and you can work against it through training habitual use of visual, auditory, and emotional perception. If doctors are trained to use these perceptive modalities in the same way with every patient, many inappropriate implicit biases can be leveled, as any incorrect, instinctive biases will be dismissed through careful observation, listening, and emotional logic.

HOW COGNITIVE BIAS APPLIES TO THE PATIENT

Almost everyone has been a patient, even if just for wellness checks. For any medical problem, analyzing patient symptoms and medical data is key to the correct diagnosis and setting up next steps, all easier said than done, particularly for complex or rare medical problems. Sometimes patient instincts are wrong; it is usually better to use logic and trust doctors. But sometimes patient instincts are correct, and healthcare providers are wrong. How can you reliably tell the difference? Ultimately, the distinction can rest on data, seeing multiple viewpoints, and having reasons for ignoring anything incongruent. Patient

"Diagnosis is not the end, but the beginning of practice."

— Martin H. Fischer, German-American Author and Physician

instincts should be balanced with the judgment of doctors.

Particularly between doctor-patient, authority bias must be taken into consideration. I have had many a polite patient smilingly shrug, *Oh, I didn't want to bother you*. I always tell them my job is to hear their skin-related concerns. If they don't alert me, I won't necessarily know. I state this as a fact with no intended snarkiness: *I cannot read minds!* Open communication, and a strong enough relationship to support that, is vital for ideal doctor-patient interactions. Doctors shouldn't be too dogmatic and yet take responsibility, recognizing the bias that authority creates – the authority figure in relationships like doctor-patient generally needs to set the right tone and space for an optimal relationship.

Getting more than one opinion is helpful because everyone has implicit bias, unique stereotyping of symptoms, categories of people, and events, a gestalt reaction that is not necessarily based on any facts but could be related to individual experience. Implicit bias affects all areas of life, at home and outside the home because heuristics help process the large amount of information encountered each day. Different doctors have different specialized areas of expertise, and specialization creates bias. Seeking out multiple opinions, particularly for difficult diagnoses in healthcare, can help overcome bias. And finally, for a physician alone to know the correct diagnosis is not enough – the knowledge and meaning of a diagnosis needs to be optimally communicated to patients. Patients have the right to ask for information and should continue to pursue the explanations they need.

PSYCHOSOCIAL DIAGNOSIS

When communicating, physicians and patients need to be able to interpret another set of data – body language, facial expressions, tone of voice, speech, and emotions. On both sides, we need to analyze and consider any barriers to proper communication between the doctor and patient, remembering that the patient is a person first. You can also teach yourself to habitually examine your own implicit bias regarding gender, race, and age. As an example, racial bias can lead to miscommunication and potentially disparate cancer outcomes in racially discordant physician-patient interactions. This is not okay. You can work against it through being more aware of what is really seen, heard, and felt and the reasons for any misperceptions.

Diagnosis doesn't just happen on a medical level between doctors and patients. You draw conclusions during all of your interactions. You may rely on known facts, but you also are prone to bias, particularly in new or complex situations. Many implicit biases have some basis in truth, but it is important to know and understand that these biases can unduly influence both doctor and patient in negative or positive ways (see **Appendix** for examples). You are making diagnoses every day in your relationships.

FOR ME: DIAGNOSIS AT WORK

My personal experience with diagnostic delay drives me to try to do better with each diagnosis that I make and communicate at work. As a physician in a field that relies greatly on visual perception, I can sometimes literally see my own cognitive bias. Because pattern recognition is key to visual analysis of a microscopic slide, I may be able to make diagnoses quickly, but I also may unknowingly ignore key information because it doesn't fit the pattern. With another look, with time, with someone else's eyes on the patient or slide, I can see where I went wrong and coach myself to not make the same mistake the next time. I talk about my mistakes to trainees, so they don't make the same ones I do. The correct diagnosis is vital.

The beauty of evaluating cognitive bias via microscopic slides is that the tissue on a slide is fixed and static. With proper tissue processing, the tissue on the slide remains the same for years. If I or someone else sees something in a slide that wasn't noted previously, that finding was always there, just not consciously perceived. I can literally see bias and error related to visual perception. In contrast, psychosocial bias is removed from the equation, because although tissue can provide clues as to skin color and age, slides themselves all look the same. From one slide to another, there is no bias of gender, social status, or other cultural differences. Diagnosis remains complex, but it is just a bit simpler in the absence of psychosocial bias.

Microscopic slides remind me of how careful I need to be once a real person is in front of me. Even when I completely forget to see the patient as a person and am thinking about medical signs and symptoms, it is not possible to interact with a patient as with a microscopic slide. Patients are not inanimate – even if I am impartial, they are forming opinions and judgments of me. Using visual perception for diagnosis of microscopic slides *and* a patient directly in front of me has taught me how much more effort is needed for me to be fully present with a patient. It makes me more aware of the psychosocial bias that I am prone to during human interaction, in addition to bias in my medical analysis. To counteract bias, I find it beneficial to ask myself if an alternative or opposite conclusion is possible, to check how others may see a situation, and to consider the biases that may be in play.

DOCTOR-PATIENT CONNECTION

A doctor is in a position of authority and should remember that patients are often looking to the doctor to set the tone of a relationship. As most people in authority also experience a flipped role (e.g. doctors may be patients themselves), both doctors and patients can know the feeling of patient powerlessness. Even though doctors are in a position of authority, patients should remember that a patient is the expert in his/her own daily, lived experience. Doctors are only human, too, and fall far short of knowing everything. What a patient may think is obvious to a doctor may not be. It is important to clearly tell the doctor, as much as is possible, about needs, concerns, and expectations. Doctors do not have all the answers, but there is a much higher chance of patients getting what they need if the doctor is aware of those needs.

KEY TAKEAWAY

Having awareness of bias is challenging, especially if you are pressed for time or if you feel you lack authority in a given situation. Habitually questioning unsubstantiated instincts, unfamiliar words, or new concepts will save both doctors and patients time as you become more able to process data more efficiently, improving the physician's ability to diagnose, both psychosocially and medically, and the patient's experience of healthcare.

PRACTICAL APPLICATIONS

Explore your implicit biases. 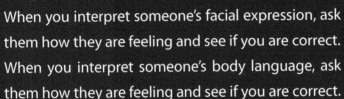https://implicit.harvard.edu/implicit/takeatest.html

Test your skills in diagnosis:
When you interpret someone's facial expression, ask them how they are feeling and see if you are correct. When you interpret someone's body language, ask them how they are feeling and see if you are correct.

Test others' skills in diagnosing/interpreting you:
When you are feeling a particular emotion (anger, disgust, fear, joy, sadness), ask someone what they think you are feeling without you saying anything. When you are feeling a particular emotion (anger, disgust, fear, joy, sadness), talk to someone on the phone and ask them what they think you are feeling based on your tone of voice as you speak.

Write a short play of a doctor-patient interaction that is relevant to you – write it as a positive interaction and, if you have time and inclination, as a negative interaction.

Act out your short play and videotape it if possible. Observe, listen, and feel emotions as you evaluate the video. What was good? What went poorly?

MY OWN IMPLICIT BIAS

I have to admit that I have a mental picture in my mind of a doctor, and it is not me. The doctor that I imagine is male, tall, Caucasian, white-haired, with bright eyes behind thin spectacles. I am of average height for a female Korean, have not yet grayed significantly, and have relatively small brown eyes and wear contact lenses. The two things I could more easily change are to wear thin spectacles and dye my hair gray!

Imposter syndrome is the feeling that you don't belong, that you don't really deserve to be where you are. I don't consciously think I have imposter syndrome, but my mental picture of a doctor tells me about my own implicit bias of what a "real" physician looks like.

If even I think that way, what about others' thought patterns? At least some do have the same bias as me, as some patients (more so in the past, when I looked younger) don't recognize me as the doctor. These patients would either call me, "Nurse" or ask me, "When is the doctor coming in?", or, "Oh, are you actually the doctor?" I knew and know they were not deliberately trying to undermine me.

FURTHER READING

87 System 1 and 2 thinking…Kahneman D. *Thinking, Fast and Slow*. New York: Farrar, Straus and Giroux, 2011.

88 "rules of thumb" or "heuristics",…Ibid.

90 Diagnosis remains fundamentally dependent on a personal interaction of a [clinician] with a patient… Kassirer JP. Imperatives, expediency, and the new diagnosis. *Diagnosis* 2014;1:11–12.

91 Physician would need to read about 29 hours/workday to keep up with medical knowledge… Alper BS, Hand JA, Elliott SG, et al. How much effort is needed to keep up with the literature relevant for primary care? *J Med Lib Assoc* 2004;92:429-437.

92 Doctors are just as biased as the rest of the human population…Dehon E, Weiss N, Jones J, Faulconer W, Hinton E, Sterling S. A systematic review of the impact of physician implicit racial bias on clinical decision making. *Acad Emer Med* 2017;24(8):895-904. AND FitzGerald C, Hurst S. Implicit bias in healthcare professionals: a systematic review. *BMC Medical Ethics* 2017;18;19. doi.org/10.1186/s12910-017-0179-8.

95 Racial bias can lead to miscommunication and potentially disparate cancer outcomes… Esnaola NF, Ford ME. Racial differences and disparities in cancer care and outcomes: Where's the rub? *Surg Oncol Clin N Am* 2012;21(3):417-viii.

98 What a patient may think is obvious to a doctor

may not be…Savitsky K, Gilovich T. The illusion of transparency and the alleviation of speech anxiety. *J Exp Soc Psychol* 2003;39:618-625.

Cognitive bias in healthcare

Croskerry P. The importance of cognitive errors in diagnosis and strategies to minimize them. *Acad Med* 2003;78(8):775-780.

O'Sullivan ED, Schofield SJ. Cognitive bias in clinical medicine. *JR Coll Physicians Edinb* 2018;48:225-232.

Busby LP, et al. Bias in radiology: The how and why of misses and misinterpretations. *Radiographics* 2018;38:236-247.

Saposnik G, et al. Cognitive biases associated with medical decisions: A systematic review. *BMC Med Inform Decis Mak* 2016;16:138.

4 DOCTOR-PATIENT CONNECTION: THINKING ABOUT HOW DOCTORS AND PATIENTS COMMUNICATE

Due to the complexity of the doctor-patient interaction, good rapport can be difficult to achieve. There have been many times, more than I would like to count or recall, when I have experienced suboptimal communication with my patients. One patient returned, in anger, just to tell me that she had tested negative for the human immunodeficiency virus (HIV). She vociferously informed me in no uncertain terms how wrong I had been. I was taken aback by her reaction as she had not said anything to me at the end of the initial visit, when I had asked her to have testing for HIV, just to be safe, as she had multiple viral lesions (termed Molluscum contagiosum). These lesions can be seen in adults, but she had many more than were typical, and acquired immunodeficiency can sometimes present this way. She had misunderstood me, believing me to be saying that she had HIV. She had been scared, shocked, and speechless but had kept quiet, saying nothing. I had not picked up on her discomfort during the first visit.

Another time, running behind on a very busy day of clinic, I briskly entered a room that had a patient that was new to me, someone I had never seen before. My medical assistant had already taken a brief history and had told me outside the room that he needed a skin examination but was not particularly concerned about anything on his skin. I greeted him as I came into the room, shook his hand, and said that I would start the skin examination. He immediately said, "Oh, you are all just business, aren't you?" I got to know him over the next couple of years (he stuck with me), and he related over time that I had seemed so "clinical" at first, so detached. Over time, he had learned that his initial impression had not been correct. I am at risk for giving the wrong first impression. My manner and my words can definitely be misinterpreted and negatively affect my doctor-patient relationships.

I am not alone in being misinterpreted. As I navigated the medical system from the time my son was nine months old, I often encountered busy clinicians, biases, and emotions that were confusing to deal with. When my son was 13 months of age and I was told that he had normal hearing, I was fully ready to accept that (and I did). My son's symptoms bothered me enough to ask the audiologist, "But is there some condition where you hear sometimes and not others?" She began walking out of the room as she said, *Oh, yes, in auditory neuropathy it can seem like hearing is fluctuating, but that is so rare!* In retrospect, she was giving me the right diagnosis in words. But her tone, manner, and body language were dismissive. Instead of trusting myself or even thinking about the diagnosis she had suggested, I mistakenly accepted her authority and her diagnosis of normal hearing, which she had given me while sitting down, earlier in the visit. Accurate communication can be difficult to achieve in healthcare, and this problem is more prevalent than anyone realizes on a day-to-day basis.

Subsequently, once my son was diagnosed as profoundly deaf due to auditory neuropathy, several of the professionals we encountered were blunt in the extreme. One said to me, *Your son acts like a deaf child.* She said this with what I perceived as a modicum of contempt – she clearly knew what a deaf child acts like, and the bald statement seemed to include the judgment that I also knew what a deaf child acts like but I had been willfully ignoring the evidence. Meanwhile, my mind began spinning at her matter-of-fact words, and I was never able to ask, *What does a deaf child act like?* Given her statement, which was uttered as absolute truth, I answered my own question internally…. *A deaf child acts like my child. This is why he touches everything. This is why he observes so carefully. This is why he ignores my voice. This is why he seems confused when routine is broken.*

He doesn't hear the words that explain what is about to happen. While I appreciated the honesty, I would have benefited from a little bit more empathy.

As a last example, as we explored the possibility of cochlear implantation, we met with several surgeons. The surgeon's bedside manner and communication skills were less important to me than his/her skill in the operating room. What becomes difficult is that it can be impossible to evaluate a surgeon's skill in the operating room – you are not there, as a family member, as a patient you are under anesthesia and not aware of what is going on, and a surgeon's behavior during a clinic visit doesn't actually have much to do with operating skill. The first surgeon we met was condescending, would not speak to me directly and instead addressed only my husband. Even so, these were not the things that made me seek another opinion. When I asked if bilateral cochlear implantation was possible for my son, instead of saying yes or no, he said, *You could find a cowboy to do it.* And quickly followed that with, *Do you want your son to have facial paralysis?* His not answering my question directly was condescending; his manner and his position of knowledge and authority made me feel uncertain and more fearful of the future. *Of course I didn't want my son to have facial paralysis!* Since I didn't get a direct answer, I obtained two more opinions. These two other surgeons both answered, *Yes! Bilateral cochlear implantation is possible.* By that time in my son's medical course, I had learned the value of getting more than one opinion. Needless to say, we didn't go with the first surgeon.

METACOGNITION TOWARD BETTER COMMUNICATION

Delivery of any message is improved by metacognitive work – thinking about how we are getting the information across. When considering how to best communicate, metaperception becomes important – it is helpful to focus on what you see, hear, and feel through body language, speech, and emotions. At the very least, you should be aware of your own body language, your speed, and the energy that you have when talking, your emotional state, and the words that you use. Mastering your speech will make you more confident, allowing you to be more persuasive and more effective in influencing and teaching others as you build relationships. Having a voice is a critical skill, just as important as collecting data and making diagnoses. You should also be aware of your conversational partner's body language, speech, and tone.

Being cognizant of these elements, including pauses, and allowing for questions are important. But most healthcare workers are pressed for time, and rushing prevents stronger relationships. Many patients are unable to voice their true concerns and feelings. Without training and knowledge, the tendency, mine included, is to be too blunt or to avoid important conversations.

DOCTORS AND COMMUNICATION

There is no standardized course that coaches medical professionals and patients how to communicate well and build strong relationships. At least, I can say that there was never such a course when I was in medical school or in training. Doctors, like most professionals, become immersed in the jargon of their field, learning an entire new language that those not in medicine often cannot comprehend. Meanwhile, communicating to patients is essential, and this important piece of being a doctor often still rests on apprenticeship, with learning in real time from those more experienced, shadowing them in their clinics, watching and learning from how they communicate. If trainees are lucky, they will see great doctor-patient relationships and learn from them.

During the initial moments of a visit, physicians need to gather data and set an agenda for the visit, and ideally there is a question to the effect of, "Anything else?" to ensure that the important concerns are captured; all concerns may not be able to be addressed, and they need to be prioritized appropriately. Dr. Larry Mauksch, a specialist in family medicine and healthcare communication, suggests that the doctor say, early in the visit, "I'd like to know if you have something else important to address today. This way you and I can figure out how to make the best use of our time."

"Speech is power: speech is to persuade, to convert, to compel."

—Ralph Waldo Emerson, American Essayist, Lecturer, Philosopher, and Poet

COMMUNICATION TIPS FROM DR. RANA AWDISH*

Tips	Potential script
DOCTOR	
Set the agenda	"…I'd like to hear what is on your mind. What brought you in today?"
Ask again	"Is there anything else?"
Explore	"What do you think is going on?" "It seems as though you are feeling [insert an emotion]. Is that true?"
Provide support	"I'll be here with you…"
Assess understanding	"How would you explain what I just told you?"
PATIENT	
Set the agenda	"What I hope to accomplish today is…" "I am hoping to learn…" "Can you explain…"
State concerns/fears	"I am worried that…"
Restate for clarity	"Can I try this in my own words?" "What I hear you saying is…"
Next steps	"How will I learn the results?"

Adapted with permission from Awdish R. Communication Tips. In: Shock: My Journey from Death to Recovery and the Redemptive Power of Hope. New York: St. Martin's Press, 2017, pp. 255-262.

PATIENTS AND COMMUNICATION

Physicians *and* patients interrupt each other. In today's world of medicine, with visits cut ever shorter, both physicians and patients often feel a time crunch. As a patient, you can and should interrupt the doctor to maximize time spent on the essentials important to you. Notably, *when* you interrupt matters; ideally, it is early on in the visit.

Patients are not always able to be up front with their doctors. Research suggests that an affirmative, *Yes*, from a patient does not actually correlate with a positive patient response. Imagine someone asking you, "Do you understand?" The tendency is to answer in the affirmative. A "yes" may only represent the fact that many women are taught to be agreeable, and many patients believe it is rude to disagree with or question a physician. A "yes" does not mean that a patient will fill a prescription or follow any recommendations. Rather than, "Yes", research suggests that an, "Oh", followed by enthusiasm is much more associated with openness to a health intervention.

This research ably demonstrates that patients do not want to contradict doctors, but patients need to realize that doctors cannot know what a patient will do if the patient only responds in the affirmative. As a patient, clear, forthright honesty is important when communicating with a doctor. If you don't understand, say so. It is okay to say, "Would you be able to repeat that?" It is even better to summarize with words like, "This is what I just heard…." If a medicine is too expensive, there may be alternatives; pharmacists can even put in requests for alternates for patients. If there is some barrier to getting to appointments or necessary treatments, patients should let doctor know. The doctor may not be able to solve it, but if the doctor doesn't even know patient concerns, it is more likely than not that those concerns will not be addressed.

METAPERCEPTION TOWARD BETTER COMMUNICATION

Courses on how to have a difficult conversation or how to create cognitive empathy can certainly help your relationships. However, not everyone has the time or means to enroll in such courses. Even if a course is taken, practice is necessary as lasting change is unlikely to develop after taking one course. Using metaperception to evaluate what you see, hear, and feel becomes useful as you can coach yourself once you start to think about doing so. You can self-model prior to having a conversation or analyze and review one that went well or poorly after the fact; existing formal programs do such analysis by focusing on what worked well, why, and creating small changes that helped promote the same. Key attributes that aid conversations are being curious, considering other perspectives, collaborating, compromising, and celebrating. Whether through a formal course or self-study, practicing communication leads to improvement.

Individual coaching by someone else can also be beneficial. Unfortunately, not everyone has access to such a coach, teacher, or mentor. I have been lucky to have had some coaching with Dr. Caruso, a pioneer in the field of emotional intelligence. He suggested catchphrases (e.g. *Tell me more.* Or *What did I miss?* Or *I'd like to return to this.*) that can be used to aid conversation. Knowledge and respect of the culture and any hierarchy is helpful. Asking questions, trying to get others to teach the point you want to emphasize, being specific about behaviors (rather than targeting a person), doing a *what if* analysis, having a go-to script for predictable situations, and teaching yourself to pause can help smooth conversations. As an example, you can teach yourself to

> "Communication is an expertise that you can learn. It resembles riding a bike or composing."
>
> — Brian Tracy, Author of *Eat that Frog*

pause, either by taking a breath or counting in your head to five or looking down for a moment. All of these actions can be taught in individual coaching and then can be implemented, practiced, and forged into habit.

COMPENSATORY PHRASES TO AID COMMUNICATION*

Tell me more.
What did I miss?
Please give me an example.
I don't see it that way.
I just happened to notice…
Let me think/reflect on that one.
I'd like to return to this.
Is there anything we can do now?
Thank you for your honesty.
I really do appreciate that.
I'm going to have to think about this.

*David Caruso, PhD, personal communication

FOR ME: COMMUNICATION AND METAPERCEPTION

I am by nature shy and introverted. Shyness and introversion are not actually the same thing, and for me the end result is that relationships do not come easy to me. While I was in school and in training, my focus was on learning necessary science, physiology, biology, pharmacology, and other subjects. Initially, as a trainee, although I interacted with patients, I was generally not the ultimately responsible physician. There was always someone senior to me who had the final say. I didn't have to battle my personality and could remain quiet in the corner.

Without fully realizing how my personality might enhance my choice of occupation, I was drawn to dermatopathology. Dermatopathology is the practice of looking at and diagnosing glass slides of patient skin disease, at a microscope, often alone. Glass slides don't have emotions or body language, and they don't talk back. My own emotions and body language are never being judged by the slides I look at. And in terms of my delivery, the vast majority of my diagnoses go out in written form on a pathology report. I can spend as much time as I want on the diagnosis and any related explanation. I can get second and third opinions on the glass slide and how to word things before I ever complete the report. Dermatopathology suits me.

Producing coherent written dermatopathology reports continues to be fun for me. I was and am interested in improving my written delivery of dermatologic diagnosis. My goal is always for my written reports to be easily understood by the physicians that read them, and starting in 2021, patients also have full, early access to those reports.

The world of dermatopathology, with less human interaction, was always a contrast with my clinical work as a dermatologist. Patients have needs and emotions, biases of their own, and they are not always transparent in what they hope to get out of the doctor-patient relationship. In a relatively short clinic visit, it can be a whirlwind to have the patient roomed, take a history, perform a comprehensive skin examination and any necessary procedures, and communicate important information to the patient. All of this action needs to be completed while being aware of the patient's questions, needs, emotions, and body language. Meanwhile, the patient is evaluating my body language, tone of voice, manner, and overall trustworthiness and competence. It is a lot. The doctor-patient relationship is very different from a doctor-inanimate glass slide interaction.

My personal experiences with miscommunication with my own patients and with the doctors that I have encountered for my own family's needs show me how much I need to improve. Because my son has cochlear implants and is profoundly deaf when he has the external portion off, I have a daily reminder of how speech and tone are not always heard, how much body language can communicate, and how a smile can be amazingly powerful.

DOCTOR-PATIENT CONNECTION: METAPERCEPTIVE COMMUNICATION

Human relations can be unpredictable. When you recognize the complexity of information that is being processed between doctor and patient, no wonder that the relationship can be fraught with difficulty. There are family, cultural, and societal rules to follow, challenges and illnesses to overcome. The mainstream culture patients are exposed to may not be the same as familial culture. The primary

DOCTOR-PATIENT COMMUNICATION   119

language of patients may not be the same as the doctor. Emotions may be expressed differently. Relationships are not easy.

But once you recognize this potential difficulty, you can do better. You can learn from your mistakes. You can change things for the next time. You can do *what-if* analyses to prepare for difficult conversations. You can strengthen your relationships.

You need to be able to accurately process the data you receive and are giving, all while instinctively using the right body language, tone, and words. Being adept takes practice – you need to form tiny habits that you can slowly capitalize into bigger ones. All this really takes is metaperception, or thinking about your perceptions – thinking about what you see, hear, and feel in a given interaction.

KEY TAKEAWAY

You can prepare the words you use, particularly if you know in advance what you need to communicate. Not only that, you can think about the best body language and tone of voice to use, to make them congruent with your words and the outcome that you want. If you are not sure, you can think back on situations that you have been in, times when communication worked well and times when it failed in your relationships. You can observe others who you think are successful in getting their message across and break down their body language, tone, and words into discrete units that you can try to emulate. Ultimately, forming habits based on what you perceive will improve your ability to deliver an accurate message, both socially and medically.

Habits are created through repetition, and the latter can be achieved through applying metaperception to what is seen, heard, and felt. **Chapters 5** to **11** of this book delve into how to do this.

"If you think too much, you fail,
because the game happens too quickly.
The key is preparation…
the data has to become instinctual."
— Joe Girardi, Manager of the New York Yankees with
> 500 Wins and the 27th World Series Championship
Title

PRACTICAL APPLICATIONS: RELATIONSHIP COMMUNICATION

Listen to yourself and others talk. Calculate how many words you speak in one minute. Listen for any pauses or filler sounds (e.g. "um").

Record yourself using your smartphone camera or your computer's camera. Watch the video and analyze your own impressions of yourself.

Hire a speech coach and meet with him/her at least four times.

Write a script for the most common difficult situation you find yourself in, during a healthcare interaction. Videotape yourself speaking in the doctor-patient (with consent) interaction – this is increasingly easy to do with built-in cameras on computers and smartphones. Evaluate your performance.

Perform what Dr. David Caruso calls "emotional what-ifs". Think about a difficult healthcare interaction. What makes communication hard? Imagine yourself talking, encountering communication barriers, and steering the conversation the right way.

FURTHER READING

108   Helpful to focus on what you see, hear, and feel… Tate P, Frame F. *The Doctor's Communication Handbook,* 8th edition. Boca Raton: CRC Press, 2019;1-142.

109   Many patients are unable to voice…Ibid.

110   "Anything else?"…Fortin AH VI, Dwamena FC, Frankel RM, Lepisto BL, Smith RC. *Smith's Patient-centered Interviewing: An evience-based method.* New York: McGraw-Hill Education, 2019.

110   "I'd like to know if…"…Mauksch LB. Questioning a Taboo: Physicians' interruptions during interactions with patients. *JAMA* 2017;317:1021-1022.

112   Affirmative, *Yes,* from a patient does not actually correlate with…Albury C, et al. GP-delivered brief weight loss interventions: A cohort study of patient responses and subsequent actions, using conversation analysis in UK primary care. *Br J Gen Pract* 2018;68:e646-e653.

114   Key attributes that aid conversations are being curious…Roddy E, Dewar B. A reflexive account on becoming reflexive: the 7 Cs of caring conversations as a framework for reflexive questioning. *Int Prac Dev J* 2016;doi:10.10.19043/IPDJ.61.008.

119   Being adept takes practice…Friesen JP, Sidhu DM, Canadas E, et al. Perceiving happiness in an intergroup context: The role of race and attention to the eyes in differentiating between true and false smiles. *J Pers Soc Psychol* 2019;116:375-395.

119 Being adept takes practice…Sheldon OJ, Dunning D, Ames DR. Emotionally unskilled, unaware, and uninterested in learning more: Reactions to feedback about deficits in emotional intelligence. *J Appl Psychol* 2014;99:125-137.

5 VISUAL PERCEPTION: FORM AN OBSERVING HABIT BY THINKING ABOUT WHAT YOU SEE, FAST AND SLOW

"It is useful to constantly observe, note, and consider."
— Leonardo da Vinci, Italian Polymath

"Christine, sometimes it's just gestalt."

This is what Dr. Ronald Barr, my first guide into the enchanting world of dermatopathology, would say to me when I would press him for reasons as to why he (always!) knew what something was. And he would also sometimes talk about so-and-so having a "good eye" for dermatopathology.

Gestalt.

A "good eye".

Both seemed infinitely mysterious.

But there is actually no secret to this. Gestalt is essentially visual recognition, and there is a number for how quickly this happens – studies have shown that visual recognition can be as quick as 50 to 200 milliseconds! *Less time than a fastball crossing home plate.* The "how" behind this rapid recognition crystallized for me through Dr. Daniel Kahneman's book, *Thinking, Fast and Slow* – near-immediate identification is System 1 thinking (see also **Chapter 2**). Dr. Kahneman uses "System 1" and "System 2" as artificial constructs of the major ways that we think – System 1 is fast processing, your intuition, your gut, *your gestalt.* System 2 is slow processing, logical, analytical, mathematical. Neither System exists; they are semantic symbols of metacognition (thinking about how we think). While neither is more reliable or precious than the other, training the brain, visually or otherwise, expands your ability to think fast.

Expert thought ultimately is System 1 thinking and develops over time. Expert thought is gestalt, and highly accurate gestalt is a marker of an expert. For my field of dermatopathology, gestalt is a "good eye". For all medical and surgical fields, gestalt is visual and cognitive recognition of the very sick patient, of critical physical examination findings, and of disease in general, as defined by deviation from health.

GESTALT RECOGNITION

You are already an expert in using this type of gestalt every day when you recognize the people around you. Facial recognition is a System 1, fast process; you have focused on the human face since you were a baby, and you are expert at immediately recognizing those familiar to you. An exception to this is if you have prosopagnosia, a disorder in which you cannot recognize faces properly, and part of this disease is related to slow cognitive processing of faces. Training (System 2 work) can improve the ability to recognize faces.

Once I started my third (and current) job in dermatopathology, this concept of "gestalt", of "just knowing", continued to simultaneously fascinate me and disturb me, much the same as religious faith. Two people in my department who have had an extraordinary impact on me, Dr. Jennifer McNiff and Dr. Jean Bolognia, each have a way of immediately perceiving things that is astounding. I could say they have the "good eye", but such words partially suggest their expertise in precise recognition of skin cancer and severe skin reactions is luck, an innate talent rather than a product of concerted effort.

A "good eye" is not just luck. There is finely honed expert instinct involved, and it is generally domain-specific – even though I can recognize skin disease more easily than a non-dermatologist can, I won't necessarily do better at other visual tasks like finding Waldo! I used to ask another one of my mentors, Dr. Earl Glusac, when I might feel gestalt. *When would I be absolutely, immediately sure of myself for a given diagnosis, even if others disagreed with me?* Earl told me such impenetrable confidence would happen with time. And he is correct – I have developed more of an instinctual "reaction" when I first view a piece of tissue under the microscope on a glass "slide". I do have such a gestalt impression for a great many slides (but not all, even now), including ones that are difficult and challenging and promote a difference of opinion among my talented group of colleagues. Expertise takes time.

So of course, I wanted to know – *how much time is needed to develop accurate gestalt?* Malcolm Gladwell, in his book *Outliers*, puts a number on expert gestalt – 10,000 hours. Meanwhile, Dr. Anders Ericsson explains that 10,000 hours is an arbitrary number; 7,500 hours may also work but the number may be closer to 20,000 hours, in terms of becoming the best in the world at something. The irony of fast thinking in an expert is how slowly such System 1 (fast) thinking develops.

Time is the factor that my mentor Dr. Earl Glusac emphasized. If we choose 10,000 hours as a starting point for expertise, we can translate that number into 20 hours/week over 10 years. Twenty hours per week, or just four hours per day in a five-day work week, may not seem like very much. But those 20 hours need to be spent in so-called deliberate practice (see **Chapter 1**).

When I think about teaching others (or myself) to recognize skin diseases, I can use this knowledge. Instant recognition means that gestalt has already developed for that particular disease. If gestalt is not there, I can consciously use System 2 to explain what needs to be observed for quick recognition. This interplay of System 1 (gestalt) and System 2 (conscious) thinking is a way to evaluate yourself and others with immediate feedback.

Dr. Daniel Kahneman's System 1 and 2 constructs shed light on the "how of visual recognition" in dermatopathology, gestalt ultimately being the development of expert, System 1 thinking. Developing visual perception into System 1 thinking does not only happen in visual specialties like dermatology and dermatopathology; visual examination of a patient is an important component of the physical examination broadly in medicine and surgery. The importance of visual perception is encoded in language. A conflict during communication may prompt someone to say something to the effect of, "I just don't see it that way." Success may be applauded with words like, "She had the vision."

Metacognition (thinking about how I see) changed my work practices. I set a goal of documenting my System 1, gestalt diagnosis for a given slide and then reviewing the slide using System 2; rattling off the data for my gestalt impression, looking for any evidence that could sway me toward a different diagnosis, consciously telling myself – I think this is X because of *1,2,3;* and it's not *Y*, which is the worst diagnosis possible, because of *4,5,6.* Any discrepancy between the diagnosis I come to using System 1 (fast) versus 2 (slow) is critiqued to arouse my brain to attention. I didn't always use metacognition, and it benefits me enormously as I am more aware of my perceptual traps and errors.

OPTICAL ILLUSIONS

Optical illusions are a fun way to approach visual recognition and metacognition. Such illusions teach you about bias and System 1 or System 2 thinking, gestalt versus rational analysis. Optical illusions demonstrate how your brain's hardwiring can trick you.

Observe the following examples.

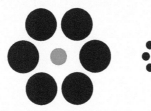

In this optical illusion, the central red circles are the same size (you can use System 2 and check for yourself with a ruler!), but visually your brain tells you the red circle on the right is larger because of the contrast with the smaller circles surrounding it (System 1, gut reaction).

Try out the Stroop effect. Test yourself with the following six boxes – for each of them, name the color of the letters.

RED   YELLOW   BLACK

PURPLE   ORANGE   BLUE

In general, naming the color of the letters is easier for the first row of boxes. For the second row, reading (System 1; fast thinking) interferes with the naming of color, and slower processing (System 2; slow thinking) is necessary to redirect the brain.

Test yourself with the story to the right. Time yourself to see how quickly you can read the story.

RUNAWAY OWEN*

Once there was a little Owen. He said, "I want to run away frm you."

"If you run away," said Mommy, "I will run after you. For you are my Owen."

"If you run after me, I will become a fireman, and I will shoot oot of the fire station so that you can't catch me."

"If you become a fireman, I will become a cowboy's rope so that I can lasso you."

"If you become a rope, then I will be an ambulnce because it looks for sick people."

"If you become an ambulance, then I will become a super fast car so that I can catch you."

"If you catch me from the super fast car, then I wll be an SUV police car and give you a ticket for speeding."

"If you gecome a police car, then I will become a police stachion so that you drive back to me."

"If you become a police station, then I will be a cannoli trck."

"If you become a cannoli truck, then I will be a berd so that I can sit on top of the truck."

"I might as well stay her and be your best friend," said Owen.

"Sure," said Mommy. "Have some cookeis!"

*In March, 2015, our auditory verbal therapist instructed us to model a story on "The Runaway Bunny" by Margaret Wise Brown, which we read all together. Our story was based on all the things he loved at the time (cannoli trucks, fire trucks).

Time yourself with the same story to see how long it takes you to proofread (can you find all 10 errors?).

Reading, a System 1 process, is fast and automatic for you over time. In contrast to reading, proofreading is a System 2, slower process. Proofreading answers: frm (from) in line 2, oot (out) in line 6, ambulnce (ambulance) in line 9, wll (will) in line 13, gecome (become) in line 15, stachion (station) in line 16, trck (truck) in line 18, berd (bird) in line 20, her (here) in line 21), cookeis (cookies) in line 23.

HOW THIS APPLIES TO DOCTORS AND PATIENTS

You may be, like me, in a field that is largely visually-oriented. You may have experienced, like me, times when you think your visual abilities or visual intelligence does not come naturally. And you may have learned, as I did, that working on an observing habit does improve visual recognition. System 2 (conscious) thinking increases your System 1 (gestalt) capability. Metacognitive work teaches you to observe more through building pattern recognition. Implementing an observing habit through use of System 1 and 2 is effective in visually-oriented fields.

Even if you are in a field that is not primarily visually-oriented, almost all doctors use vision in the physical examination, and all patients are also observers of their own healthcare encounters. Learning to observe is beneficial.

Visual perception is a broad intelligence. Your visual sense communicates to you not only diagnosis (especially for those like me, in visual medical specialties) but also critical information. A patient's general appearance can give important clues to overall health; an inverted nipple can be a sign of breast cancer. In baseball, accurate pitch recognition allows for more accuracy in hitting the ball. In football, basketball, and soccer, having a well-developed sense of where everyone is on the field, court, or pitch makes a better player.

Spatial ability is part of visual intelligence as well. When I first spoke with Dr. David Caruso, an expert in emotional intelligence, he used an analogy to explain how we can overcome some deficits in emotional intelligence. If I was low in spatial ability, if he gave me detailed directions on how to find his office, I could follow them (using System 2 thinking), with practice, but I might lose my way once or twice or more. Instead, a global positioning system (GPS) would save me time. I wouldn't have to think about how to get to his office; I could rely on the GPS. But also note that, as would be true for most people, once I've followed the GPS a certain number of times (and this number may vary for different people), I won't need the machine anymore, for at least that one task of getting to Dr. Caruso's office. Over time, the GPS would teach me a pattern through continuous feedback on the correct way to get there. The GPS is a useful tool due to the real-time feedback along the way that can coach me and reroute me. A GPS is a particular method to get to the right place.

Intelligently using visual perception is like a GPS. Creating an observing habit will benefit you and create road maps that you can habitually use. Observing carefully is an ability that can become a well-traveled, familiar road that you can take with ease.

Amy Herman, the author of *Visual Intelligence: Sharpen Your Perception, Change Your Life*, hosts professional development seminars where participants use art to increase observational powers. Her idea originated after she had observed the Workshop on Observational Skills at Yale Medical School, a first-year medical student course. The workshop had been designed by Dr. Irwin Braverman, Professor of Dermatology, and

"Picture your brain forming new connections as you meet the challenge and learn."
— Carol Dweck, PhD, Psychologist and Author of *Mindset: The New Psychology of Success*

Linda Friedlaender, Head of Education at the Yale Center for British Art. Dr. Braverman noticed that over the years, all medical trainees benefited from honing their observational skills by describing art at a museum. Since that original course, it has been shown that increasing visual literacy benefits those in careers ranging from medicine to finance to government.

FOR ME: VISUAL PERCEPTION

Learning to consciously use System 1 and System 2 in my analysis of microscopic slides and skin examinations – this double-check generated more detailed visual data that I could ultimately use for diagnosis. Using both systems of thought makes me a better doctor and educator, helping me to design appropriate research, education, and treatment plans.

In training myself to observe skin disease and through learning to see what my colleagues can sometimes see but I initially cannot, I developed an observing habit at work. I realized that this habit did not automatically transfer to other domains, and I could consciously apply it beyond microscopic slides and skin examinations. I could teach myself to observe more during patient interactions, to better appreciate the unique person in front of me as well as my own reactions. I could improve my teaching by observing students and residents, checking for signs of engagement or confusion, including my own impact. Rather than having blinders on to the rich visual information around me, I wondered, *What would happen if I used an observing habit in my daily life?*

DOCTOR-PATIENT CONNECTION: AN OBSERVING HABIT IS A SKILL

System 1 and System 2 thinking affect your perception of everything around you, with optical illusions being tangible examples. Because most of us use vision every day, images are constantly being processed every waking moment. Even with your eyes closed, you can picture

"...everyone can change and grow through application and experience."
—Carol Dweck, PhD, Psychologist

something in your "mind's eye." When you harness System 1 and System 2 processing, you will tend to get more accurate visual information, and just as metacognition helps me analyze what a microscopic slide is telling me, using both Systems can do the same for healthcare interactions.

Vision is powerful. Literally looking in a certain direction changes your body position enough that you will steer yourself that way, even if you are headed for a crash. I always doubt this phenomenon, which I notice the most when snowboarding or biking – and then every time I look at something and think, "I don't want to crash into that!" almost always, I will crash. Because that's where I was looking. If I look instead toward where I actually want to go, the crash is preventable. Your gaze controls your destination.

KEY TAKEAWAY

Even if you continue to think that visual information is not essential for you, tweaking just one small thing in what you observe can help prove that you can augment visual capability; you can see yourself change (no pun intended). Importantly, for something to become habit, you have to care enough about and work for change. Performing the exercises at the end of this chapter may not be something you will be passionate about or something that will necessarily change your life for the better. However, they are simple observations that can prove to you that you can manipulate your visual intelligence. Seeing "fast" can be developed by "slow" conscious observation. The more you work at noticing certain details, those details are recognized "faster" and more easily, eventually with hardly any effort. You can learn an observing habit with time, constructive feedback, and deliberate practice.

"Learn to see, learn to hear, learn to feel, learn to smell, and know that by practice alone you can become expert."
—William S. Thayer, MD, Professor of Clinical Medicine, Johns Hopkins Hospital

PRACTICAL APPLICATIONS: AN OBSERVING HABIT

Consider how you use your vision on a daily basis. How important is an observing habit in what you do?

Visit an art museum and spend at least five minutes observing a work of art before reading the title and any other information.

Look at Salvador Dalí's art at a museum or online. Observe the double/multiple images that may be seen.

Consciously note the eye color of five people a day for a five-day period.

Consciously note three items of clothing on three people a day for a five-day period.

Consciously note one thing about the body language of a person for a five-day period.

ARTISTS AND VISUAL PERCEPTION

All art is a rendering of the world as perceived by an artist. Great artists are able to make you see the world differently, perhaps because artists likely do not see the world the same way as nonartists. Studies have shown that nonartists tend to focus on objects in a scene, while artists look at color, shading, and lines, spending less time on actual objects. While a slight difference in the perspective of each eye helps to render a feeling of three dimensions to the two-dimensional images "seen" by the eye, artists are *more* likely to be unable to re-create three-dimensionality, which is called stereoblindness. Stereoblindness could be considered a disability, but it likely aids artists in their craft – they literally see the world differently.

How you see things can be affected by color. Color can literally set the tone. Red generally signifies danger or anger but also love and passion, while yellow may do so as well or be linked to calmness. Purple signifies mystery, pink innocence, green renewal if vibrant and monotony if dull, and blue isolation or wonder. Color influences you.

While color manipulates you in a subliminal

fashion, the human face is what you are most consciously drawn to look at. The human eye is trained to look at faces from babyhood. Filmmakers take advantage of this obsession with faces, and about 90% of shots in popular movies include the face of a character. When filmmakers want the viewer to pay attention, they often use close-up shots of a face, especially centering on the face and eyes. Artists often concentrate on the human face as well.

Part of the purpose of art is to show things in new ways. Artists alter perception to surprise you or generate other emotions. Examining art can strengthen your ability to observe.

SALVADOR DALI: DOUBLE/MULTIPLE IMAGES

Salvador Dalí was a well-known Spanish Surrealist artist who often included double/multiple imagery in his art. He masterfully demonstrated that what you see is constructed by the brain. What you see as "reality is the product of the habits of the mind, more than of the eye". His intent was for you to challenge reality and see more.

An illusion can be defined as the "disconnect

between physical reality and subjective perception". In a visual illusion, you may perceive something that is not there, or ignore something that is there, or perceive something differently than reality. Illusions are concrete examples of how the brain can deceive you.

The human eye can only produce a high-resolution image for just 10% of any given visual field, but you see all that is around you in high-definition through complex neural processing. The brain is skilled at completing images for you and creating a three-dimensional construct from two-dimensional vision. Dalí's double/multiple image capitalizes on this brain skill.

"[My art] tangibly
makes the very world of
delirium
pass to the level of
reality."
— Salvador Dalí, Spanish Painter

FURTHER READING

126 Visual recognition can be as quick as 50 to 200 milliseconds...Caharel S, et al. Face familiarity decisions take 200 msec in the human brain: Electrophysiological evidence from a go/no-go speeded task. *J Cogn Neurosci* 2014;26:81-95.

126 The "how" behind this rapid recognition crystallized...Kahneman D. *Thinking, Fast and Slow*. New York: Farrar, Straus and Giroux, 2011.

127 Since you were a baby...Mardo E, et al. Adults' markers of face processing are present at age 6 and are interconnected along development. *Perception* 2018;47:1002. AND Bank S, et al. Face and body recognition show similar improvement during childhood. *J Exp Child Psychol* 2015;137:1. AND Jeffery L, et al. Insights into the development of face recognition mechanisms revealed by face after effects. *Br J Psychol* 2011;102:799.

127 Part of this disease is related to slow cognitive processing of faces...Towler J, et al. The cognitive and neural basis of developmental prosopagnosia. *Q Exp Psycho* (Hove) 2017;70: 316.

127 Can improve the ability to recognize faces... Corrow SL, et al. Training face perception in developmental prosopagnosia through perceptual learning. *Neuropsychologia* 2019;134:107196.

128 Necessarily do better at other visual tasks like finding Waldo...Sheridan H, et al. The holistic processing account of visual expertise in medical image perception: A review. *Front Psychol* 2017;8:1620.

129 A number on expert gestalt – 10,000 hours... Gladwell M. *Outliers: The story of success.* New York: Little, Brown and Company, 2008.

129 Dr. Anders Ericsson explains that 10,000 hours is an arbitrary number...Ericsson A, Pool R. Peak: Secrets from the new science of expertise. Boston: Houghton Mifflin Harcourt, 2016. AND Robert Pool, Anders Ericsson, https://www.salon.com/2016/04/10/malcolm gladwell got us wrong our research was key to the 10000 hour rule but heres what got oversimplified/

130 System 1 and System 2...Kahneman D. *Thinking, Fast and Slow.* New York: Farrar, Straus and Giroux, 2011.

Stroop effect...Stroop JR. Studies of interference in serial verbal reactions. *J Exp Psychol* 1935;18(6):643-662.

134 Reading vs. proofreading...Shafto MA. Proofreading in young and older adults: The effect of error category and comprehension difficulty. *Int J Environ Res Public Health* 2015;12:14445-14460.

136 Amy Herman, the author of...Herman A. *Visual Intelligence: Sharpen Your Perception, Change Your Life.* New York: Houghton Mifflin Harcourt, 2016.

137 Dr. Braverman noticed that over the years... Braverman IM. To see or not to see: how visual training can improve observational skills. *Clin*

Dermatol 2011;29(3):343-346.

137 It has been shown that increasing visual literacy...Goodman TR, Kelleher M. Improving novice radiology trainees' perception using fine art. *J Am Coll Radiol* 2017;14(10):1337-1340. AND Dolev JC, Friedlaender LK, Braverman IM. Use of fine art to enhance visual diagnostic skills. *JAMA* 2001;286:1020-1021.

139 Your gaze controls your destination...Authie CN, Hilt PM, N'Guyen S, Berthoz A, Bennequin D. Differences in gaze anticipation for locomotion with and without vision. *Front Hum Neurosci* 2015;doi.org/10.3389/fnhum.2015.00312. AND Jacob MS, Duffy CJ. Steering transforms the cortical representation of self-movement from direction to destination. *J Neurosci* 2015;35:16055-16063.

143 Reality is the product of the habits of the mind, more than of the eye...Martinez-Conde S, Conley D, Hine H, Kropf J, Tush P, Ayala A, Macknik SL. Marvels of illusion: Illusion and perception in the art of Salvador Dalí. *Front Hum Neurosci* 2015:9:496.

143 Disconnect between physical reality and subjective perception...Martinez-Conde S, Macknik SL. The neuroscience of illusion. *Sci Am Spec Rep* 2010;20:4-7.

144 "tangibly makes the very world of delirium pass to the level of reality". Finkelstein H. Salvador Dalí: Double and Multiple Images. *American Imago* 1983;40:311-335.

6 VISUAL DATA FOR OPTIMIZING HEALTHCARE INTERACTIONS

I remember clearly, because the same thing would happen so often and yet I never fully understood the meaning in the moment, how my chubby 18-month-old son, perched on my hip, would turn my face toward his, pulling gently on my chin. If I was wearing sunglasses and he could not see my eyes, sometimes he would also take hold of the frames and push them up to reveal my eyes, searching my face. I would smile at him, saying words that he likely could not hear (well), given his deafness which was not diagnosed till later. I was unaware at the time that his desire to see my eyes and face were necessary for him to understand me.

I am grateful that I remember smiling. That I remember well, because he would grin back in return, his pudgy cheeks folding upward. These moments are imprinted in memory, mainly because receiving that smile in return was so rewarding. My body language being mirrored back to me – I learned this lesson through my son. I still treasure the feeling of connecting, through eye contact, shared smiles, and a deliberate pause.

BODY LANGUAGE NUTS AND BOLTS

Body language (including facial expression, covered in **Chapter 10**) is a key component of communication, including in healthcare interactions. Body language is key to connecting, to likeability or charisma, and patients want to like their medical professionals. When patients like their doctors, it is easier for the doctors and patients to connect. Charismatic body language strengthens healthcare relationships by generating trust and confidence. Importantly, charismatic body language can be developed into habit.

In terms of charisma, a certain amount of eye contact is important, not 100% of the time and not 0% of the time. In the US, a "safe zone" of about 30-50% is useful to aim for; in other words, about one-third to one-half of the time you are talking to another person, or speaking in front of a larger audience, you should make eye contact. Once I thought about eye contact, I became more conscious of what I actually do. I audited myself and realized that, in general, when speaking, I rarely would make eye contact! This is exacerbated by the electronic medical record, as I have to type and click while looking at the computer screen rather than the patient's face.

My lack of making eye contact is also possibly a consequence of my cultural upbringing – a large part of my youth was spent in South Korea, where well-behaved girls were demure, with a downward gaze. Before I understood the value of eye contact, I didn't keep my eyes downcast, but I often looked everywhere possible other than at the people listening to me. This behavior is not ideal, and eye contact should not be avoided in mainstream American culture.

Once you can establish eye contact, you have to remember to pause. According to Zoe Chance, a charismatic speaker, author, and professor in the Yale School of Management, people don't listen during speech; they listen during silence. While the brain is encoding speech, the brain cannot also begin to comprehend that information. Pausing creates the space to listen, and yet many of us try to avoid silence because we are inherently uncomfortable with it.

In addition to a verbal pause, when you are introduced or introduce yourself, you should also pause with your body, holding yourself still for a moment in time, in what Zoe Chance terms a bask. You can also bask when complimented or applauded. I have often seen professionals, children, and others have difficulty accepting a simple compliment (myself included). You need to bask, using a moment's stillness, and everyone connects.

Zoe Chance's "shine" is another concept that can be used one-on-one or in a larger group setting to build charisma. Depending on your personality, shining may be harder or easier in either situation. "Shining" is connecting, on some level, through body language or other means. In part, the act relates to taking up more space, analogous to raising your arms in victory, which is a sign of pride that crosses cultures. When you take up more space, you command attention. To catch someone's interest, you can make eye contact, lean or walk toward someone, make a commanding gesture. Shining is confidence and helps build charisma.

In contrast to a good amount of eye contact, pausing, basking, and shining, certain gestures can discredit you and prevent a good connection between doctor and patient. You may fidget, put your hands in your pockets, slouch, tap, jiggle a pen,

ZOE CHANCE:* TOWARD CHARISMA

Make eye contact

Pause (deliberately allow for silence)

Bask (consciously hold yourself still for a moment)

Shine (connect to your audience, e.g. through walking toward an audience member)

*Assistant Professor in the Yale School of Management

twirl hair, scratch, cough or otherwise clear your throat. You may be too rigid. These self-comforting gestures often indicate discomfort. When you feel shame or humility, you might contract your body smaller, a mostly cross-cultural, universal reaction. Before you can pinpoint the meaning of an individual's gestures, you need to know his/her baseline, and this can be hard in the relatively short healthcare interaction, especially in an initial visit. Body language sends a message out to the world, and it may be misinterpreted. With careful observation and practice, we can become more accurate at decoding body language.

DRESS CODE NUTS AND BOLTS

In addition to body language, which can be positive or negative, particularly when we meet others for the first time, general appearance (including hair, makeup, clothing, accessories) is an important part of the visual impression. Studies have shown that appearance matters and can have direct effects on perceived competence. We evaluate others (more or less) on their general appearance, yet many (including me) do not carefully consider how appearance changes how we ourselves are perceived.

Mode of dress has an effect on healthcare interactions, and this is evident in the typical garb associated with patients and doctors – the patient gown and the white coat. Less has been written about the patient gown, but it is a symbol of lower status and decreased agency – it is generic, ill-fitting, impersonal, undignified, and unattractive.

In contrast, the white coat has a fair amount written about it in medical literature. Studies over the past several decades have shown that patients prefer doctors who wear the traditional white coat. Although I knew the importance of the white coat, for a several-year period, I saw patients without wearing a white coat over my street clothes. I somewhat unconsciously desired that my choice of clothing should have no bearing on the care I delivered. However, as an Asian female physician who looks relatively young, for better or worse, wearing the white coat instantly gives me a degree of authority and recognition that simply isn't automatically there without a white coat. An implicit bias – an unconscious bias – comes along with the white coat; the bias is a positive one that helps establish the doctor-patient relationship.

Once I realized the importance of the white coat, I began to wear it again. The white coat is gender neutral and is recognized as the garb of a physician. It seemed foolish to not take advantage of a positive implicit bias. Dressed in a white coat, I am more easily recognized as a doctor. Once I realized the difference the coat made in how my patients perceived and responded to me, I easily achieved the measurable goal of wearing my white coat 100% of the time when I would see patients. The white coat is a type of uniform that aids people's recognition of a role.

As the patient gown can be so impersonal, I also try to at least greet patients and make our introductions before the patient changes into the patient gown. If we have a fair amount to talk about after the skin examination, I will try to take the time to step out so that they can dress before we discuss important matters. Seeing a patient in their own clothes, rather than a gown, gives clues to their personality and is a reminder of their unique personhood.

METAPERCEPTION IN OBSERVING

Body language and appearance convey messages

and can either replace or enhance spoken words. Body language in particular, so important for my son in his interpretation of me, is important in doctor-patient connection. Body language affects how people are perceived, and importantly, your own body language affects you. Most do not think to consciously control body language, but becoming aware of body language is advantageous.

You need to check your own body language, your instinctive interpretation of others' body language, and a conscious assessment of potential cultural factors involved. When you greet others, you need to be aware of potential cultural differences and what is appropriate for a particular situation. Smiling and open body language are generally appreciated cross-culturally; eye contact, touch, and hand gestures are more likely to have culture-specific meanings. In traditional Korean culture, handshakes are less preferred and bowing, particularly to elders and those in authority, is the norm. Just as the firmness of a handshake can vary, the depth of a bow can vary and potentially signify the level of respect that is proffered. For the culturally unaware, a handshake or a bow may be woefully misconstrued. Just as

"The body never lies."
— Martha Graham, American
Modern Dancer and
Choreographer

a handshake can be misinterpreted across cultures, hand gestures are also not universal. A thumbs up in the US is a good thing, but in the Middle East, it is potentially a curse. Mirroring others in body language can be important for optimal connection, and cultural context can be critical for appropriate interpretation of body language and mode of dress. Accurate perception is important as we pursue optimal doctor-patient connection.

KEY TAKEAWAY

Observation is important in the doctor-patient interaction, not only for doctors to make a clinical diagnosis but also for doctor-patient communication and connection. Eye contact is helpful in establishing connection, as what you focus on signals what is important to you. Observed facial expressions, body language, and appearance are factors in nonverbal communication.

CREATING AN OBSERVING HABIT FOR DOCTOR-PATIENT CONNECTION

DOCTOR

Start with noting the eye color (see **Introduction**) of each patient as you enter the room. This will create a habit of eye contact and make the patient (rather than the electronic medical record or something else) your focus.

Try to set an example of positive body language that the patient can mirror back to you – examples include smiling as you greet the patient by name, sitting and gently leaning toward the patient, facing the patient as much as possible, sharing the electronic medical record screen with the patient, and using your gaze and body position to engage the patient.

PATIENT

It is human nature to mirror others' body language – as the patient, you can try to redirect the doctor by making eye contact with the doctor, smiling, or deliberately using the body language that you want to see in your doctor.

PRACTICAL APPLICATIONS: OBSERVING

What kind of body language do you commonly notice?

What is the dress code at work or other situations you find yourself in? Assess your own mode of dress and check if you are an outlier or if you generally conform. Consider the balance between authenticity and conformity.

Consider requests during a heathcare interaction – what facial expressions, posture, gestures are most or least effective, in your view?

How does what patients or doctors are wearing affect the interaction?

"We don't know
where our first impressions come from
or precisely what they mean, so we don't
always appreciate
their fragility."
— Malcolm Gladwell, Canadian Author, Journalist,
and Public Speaker

SIGNED LANGUAGE VERSUS BODY LANGUAGE AND EXPRESSIONS

Signed language provides an opportunity to think about the true role of body language and facial expressions in communication. Signed language is more than just hand gestures, not just pantomime – like any spoken language, signed language has rules of grammar and syntax and structure, encoded by hand, face, and body movements rather than spoken words (see **Chapter 8**). The entire body is involved, as are particular linguistic facial expressions. Proscribed movements of the arm, torso, head, and parts of the face can encode grammatical signals as well as indication of a question, statement, or command. Such movements are part of signed language and necessary for proper communication, in contrast to spoken language, where meaning can be altered by, but is not dependent on, facial expressions or body language.

Certain gestures related to body language can have some similarity to encoded gestures that have proscribed meaning in signed language, and particular facial expressions related to emotion can have resemblance to encoded facial expressions of signed language. For example, raising the eyebrows indicates a question in American Sign Language. Across cultures, the emotional facial expression of surprise also has momentarily raised eyebrows. Despite this overlap, signed language and body language, including emotional facial expressions, are processed by the brain differently.

Signed and spoken language are both primarily processed in language centers in the left side of the brain. There are 2 major areas of the left side of the brain involved in language, termed Broca's and Wernicke's areas. Broca's has a major function in production of language, either signed or spoken; Wernicke's in the perception and understanding of language, either signed or spoken.

In contrast to signed and spoken language, emotions, including emotional facial expressions, are processed on the right side of the brain, in both users of signed and spoken language. Voice prosody, which conveys emotion in spoken language, is also processed in the right brain. Ultimately, on a neural level, facial expressions and gestures do not have the same encoded meaning as signed language.

FURTHER READING

150 Body language is a key component of communication...Tipper CM, Signorini G, Grafton ST. Body language in the brain: constructing meaning from expressive movement. *Front Hum Neurosci* 2015;9:450. AND Martin L, DiMatteo M. Clinical interactions. In: Hall J, Knapp M, eds. *Nonverbal Communication*. Boston, MA: De Gruyter Mouton, 2013:833-858.

151 A certain amount of eye contact is important... Brooks CI, Church MA, Fraser L. Effects of duration of eye contact on judgments of personality characteristics. *J Soc Psychol* 1986;126. AND Gorawara-Bhat R, Cook M. Eye contact in patient-centered communication. *Patient Educ Couns* 2011;82:442. AND Riess H, Kraft-Todd G. E.M.P.A.T.H.Y.: A tool to enhance nonverbal communication between clinicians and their patients. *Acad Med* 2014;89:1108-1112.

152 People don't listen during speech...https://hbr.org/2015/05/if-you-want-people-to-listen-stop-talking
Pausing creates the space to listen...https://medium.com/@3cenglish.tutorial/the-power-of-pause-in-conversations-dce26777ce20

152 Zoe Chance terms a bask...Chance, Z. *Influence for Nice People: The New Science of Making More Friends, Money, Impact--and Joy*. Random House, 2022.

152 Zoe Chance's "shine"...Ibid.

153 Raising your arms in victory, which is a sign of pride...https://www.nytimes.com/2008/09/02/

health/02prid.html AND Tracy JL, Matsumoto D. The spontaneous expression of pride and shame: Evidence for biologically innate nonverbal displays. *PNAS* 2008;105(33):11655-11660.

153 Building charisma per Zoe Chance...Chance, Zoe. *Influence for Nice People: The New Science of Making More Friends, Money, Impact, and Joy.* Random House, 2022.

153 Certain gestures can discredit you...Hall JA, et al. Nonverbal behavior in clinician-patient interaction. *Appl Prev Psychol* 2002;4:21-37. AND Silverman J. Doctors' non-verbal behavior in consultations: look at the patient before you look at the computer. *Br J Gen Pract* 2010;60:76-68.

154 Might contract your body smaller...Tracy JL, Matsumoto D. The spontaneous expression of pride and shame: Evidence for biologically innate nonverbal displays. *PNAS* 2008;105(33):11655-11660.

155 The patient gown...Wellbery C, Chan M. White coat, patient gown. *Med Humanit* 2014;40:90-96.

155 The white coat...Ibid. AND Petrilli CM, Saint S, Jennings JJ, Caruso A, Kuhn L, Snyder A, Chopra V. Understanding patient preference for physician attire: a cross-sectional observational study of 10 academic medical centres in the USA. *BMJ Open* 2018;8(5):e021239.

156 White coat is gender neutral and is recognized as the garb of a physician...Rehman SU, et al.

What to wear today? Effect of doctor's attire on the trust and confidence of patients. *Am J Med* 2005;118:1279-1286. AND Lill MM, et al. Judging a book by its cover: descriptive survey of patients' preferences for doctors' appearance and mode of address. *BMJ* 2005;331:1524-1527. AND McKinstry B, et al. Putting on the style: what patients think of the way their doctor dresses. *Br J Gen Pract* 1991;41:275-278. AND Chung H, et al. Doctor's attire influences perceived empathy in the patient-doctor relationship. *Patient Educ Couns* 2012;89:387-389. AND Douse J, et al. Should doctors wear white coats? *Postgrad Med J* 2004;80:284-286.

157 Body language and appearance convey messages...Mehrabian A, Wiener M. Decoding of inconsistent communications. *Journal of Personality and Social Psychology* 1967:6: 109–114. AND Mehrabian A, Ferris SR. Inference of Attitudes from Nonverbal Communication in Two Channels". *Journal of Consulting Psychology* 1967;31:248-252. AND Pease B, Pease A. *The Definitive Book of Body Language: The Hidden Meaning Behind People's Gestures and Expressions.* Bantam, 2006. AND Sokolov AA, et al. Gender affects body language reading. *Front Pscyhol* 2011;2:16. AND Carney DR, et al. Review and summary of research on the embodied effects of expansive (vs. contractive) noverbal displays. *Psychol Sci* 2015;26:657-663.

157 Potential cultural differences...LaFrance M, Mayo C. Cultural aspects of nonverbal communication. *Int J Intercul Rel* 1978;2:71-89. AND Juckett G.

Cross-cultural medicine. *Am Fam Physician* 2005;72:2267-2274.

157 To have culture-specific meanings...Lorié A, Reinero DA, Phillips M, Zhang L, Riess H. Culture and nonverbal expressions of empathy in clinical settings: A systematic review. *Patient Educ Couns* 2017;100:411-424.

162 Signed and spoken language are both primarily processed in language centers...Campbell R, et al. Sign language and the brain: A review. *The Journal of Deaf Studies and Deaf Education* 2008;13:3-20.

162 Emotions, including emotional facial expressions, are processed on the right side of the brain...Newman AJ, et al. Neural systems supporting linguistic structure, linguistic experience, and symbolic communication in sign language and gestures. *Proc Natl Acad Sci USA* 2015;112:11684-11689. AND Kolod E. How does learning sign language affect perception? *Intel Science Talent Search* 2004;http://psych.nyu.edu/pelli/#intel

7 AUDITORY PERCEPTION: FORM A LISTENING HABIT BY THINKING ABOUT WHAT YOU HEAR, FAST AND SLOW

"We have two ears and one mouth so that we can listen twice as much...."
— Epictetus, Greek Philosopher

I had always taken listening somewhat for granted; this cavalier attitude came to a jarring stop once my son was diagnosed at age two with deafness. We chose cochlear implantation, even though for him we were told that cochlear implants were unlikely to give him access to sound, because there were no other medical options. For his particular diagnosis, auditory neuropathy, there was little evidence that the cochlea was the biologic, underlying cause of his auditory neuropathy. If he had a problem in his cochlea, cochlear implants would help him. If his problem was past the cochlea, for example, in the nerves going from the cochlea to the brain, cochlear implants would not change his ability to hear. What we did know from imaging studies of my son's ears and brain was that he had an abnormal layout inside his ears, possibly extending into and affecting his brain. His anatomy was somewhat obscured on radiologic studies, but one of the nerves important for hearing looked a bit abnormally thin. If that was the case, cochlear implants wouldn't fix the size of that nerve, and they wouldn't bring sound to the brain. Cochlear implantation was a last resort in my son's case that was potentially going to be ineffective in giving him adequate access to sound; the experts told me that his prognosis for acquiring age-matched spoken language was poor.

Even though there were very early reports of engineering artificial structures of the ears, a bionic ear was still more science fiction than present day. For the ability to listen to develop, there must be access to sound; there is a point of no return, where, despite the plasticity of the brain, necessary connections cannot develop properly. Most experts considered that critical age to be around five years; since he was two, I felt we only had a three-year span of time to work with. More than ever, I wished for advances in science to riot the world. I hoped for doctors and scientists to break down the walls of current knowledge and techniques with new and better options.

While I could dream, we had to have a practical plan for the present, using the current choices and technologies available. And even though I was told that they might not work for my son and his particular diagnosis and layout of his inner ears, cochlear implants and auditory verbal therapy (AVT) were the recommended path to achieve spoken language. Today, many don't think my son is deaf because AVT guided the steps toward listening and spoken language.

I had never heard of AVT before we needed to use it, and you may think that AVT has no relevance to you. It probably doesn't, in terms of speech and language acquisition, if you have typical hearing. The applicability of AVT is that it teaches how to create habit (a System 1 process, see **Chapter 2**), something everyone benefits from.

In AVT, parents are crucial teachers, as evidenced by the six principles that are family-based – parents and therapists must work together (see **Appendix**). Statistically, only about 13% of a child's life is spent in formal education by age 18, meaning that a whopping 87% of a child's time is outside of school. These hours are a very important source of learning. Furthermore, in most countries, the school year is no more than 75% of a child's year. If any school-based therapy is not somehow continued during the summer, a full one-fourth or more of the year is lost in terms of therapeutic intervention. If you bring therapy into the home, as a part of daily life, there will be five-plus hours a day of therapy just counting the hours from three to eight pm. Parents and caregivers have a critical role in AVT, in their child's education.

Similarly, even for the majority of doctors, hours at home outnumber work hours. If principles of observing and listening are maximized outside of work, there is vastly increased opportunity to work on improving interpersonal connections. If you are already a great listener outside of healthcare interactions, it may just take resetting your mental view of a healthcare appointment in order to change it for the better – make a conscious effort to build a healthcare relationship the way you would any other meaningful connection.

As a patient-centered, home-based method, AVT teaches a listening habit, over the long-term creating System 1, "fast" listening via controlled use of System 2, "slow" analysis (see **Chapters 1** and **3**). If one hears that the "s" at the end of a plural word is dropped, one completes tasks to emphasize that "s" in as natural a way as possible, using AVT techniques. Tasks are all conscious and measurable, building on each other to slowly create language patterns in the brain that become rote and part of System 1 ("fast") listening.

The brilliance of AVT is that it maximizes the natural ability of the brain to forge connection. Through focus and repetition (System 2 work), habit is borne in the brain, and habits are System 1, "fast" processing, used easily without conscious effort. Some principles of AVT (see **Appendix** to learn more) that are of use to anyone interested in improving communication are 1) optimal results are a result of strong partnerships between healthcare professionals and patients/families, 2) therapy cannot be only clinic-based, and therapy must be able to be continued and reinforced in daily home life, 3) measurable goals (see **Appendix**) are set over discrete time intervals; once goals are reached, new goals are set, and 4) the goal of AVT is to create a listening habit – to create the habit of asking, *What did I hear*? A similar listening habit can be applied to critical healthcare interactions, where partnerships between doctors and patients are important, particularly for diagnoses and treatments that affect a given patient's daily life.

AUDITORY ILLUSIONS

There is an amazing breadth and depth of auditory perception. Just as optical illusions teach you about the brain's representations of visual reality, auditory illusions do the same for auditory reality. As such illusions are dependent on sound, it is not possible to fully demonstrate them in written form. However, if you think of an illusion as imagining something that is not there, people experience illusory sound to varying degrees with the written word. Auditory perception can be manipulated.

Comic books and poetry can be used as examples of perceived sound that is not truly heard.
Consider the following:

POW!   **POOOOOWWWWW!!!!**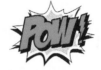

When you read the three letters above, you may "hear" the words in your head. There are "rules", with larger letters representing louder sounds and repetition of letters correlating with duration (time). Jagged, sharp lines also produce emphasis. With experience with comic books, certain sounds also become associated intuitively with a certain character or event – for example, the "SNIKT" that correlates with Wolverine's claws appearing in the comic *X-Men*. Sounds can be encoded in words, on a phonetic basis but also related to repetition and appearance.

The Rain Falls Down

The rain falls down drop by drop
Watch the rain fall as at a stop.
Want to read a book?
Or do a puzzle?
Or want to do some art?
No, I want to watch the rain
instead of reading
or doing a puzzle
or having a snack.
I want to watch the rain,
pretty drop by drop.`
The rain falls down.

The Rain Falls Down

The rain falls   drop by
drop
           down

Watch the rain fall as at a
stop.

Want to read a book?
Or do a puzzle?
Or want to do some art?

No, I want to watch the rain
instead of reading
or doing a puzzle
or having a snack.
I want to watch the rain,
pretty drop by drop.
The rain falls d
             o
               w
                n.

This poem was written by my daughter when she was in first grade. The words are exactly the same on the left versus the right. On the right side, the arrangement of the words causes a difference in the way the poem is "hear"d, regardless of whether the poem is read aloud or silently. Spaces between words and letters create silence.

"There's a lot of difference between listening and hearing."

—GK Chesterton, British Author and Journalist

HOW THIS APPLIES TO DOCTORS AND PATIENTS

The success of AVT is predicated on hard work, daily challenges, and individualized feedback that ultimately create a listening habit. I had never heard of AVT before learning that my son was deaf; there are very few (not even 1000) professionals in the United States certified in AVT. Given it is such a small field, and very few people have access to it (we were lucky), you may wonder why you even need to know about it. What does it have to do with you?

The importance of AVT lies in its basic methodology – it is based in the home, in daily life. AVT is not possible without connection to a patient's family, and it is through AVT that I began to comprehend how a treatment plan changes based on knowing the unique circumstances and home life of a patient, while having expertise in exactly what needs to be done to achieve a desired outcome. In other words, my son's auditory verbal therapist could see my son, and me, in the lived experience of our own world; she knew our home life because while half of our therapy sessions were at her workplace, the other half were either at my son's daycare or in our home. Doctors today almost never know patients in that way, and it is to the detriment of optimal diagnosis and care. But doctors used to – compare a doctor who makes house calls or a doctor who practices in a small town as a family practitioner and sees an entire family over decades to a doctor practicing in an urban, academic setting seeing a new patient for the first time, for 15 minutes. It will be much harder for the latter physician to scratch the surface of who a patient is.

Compounding this problem of increased distance (literally and figuratively) between doctors and patients, we are all selectively deaf – we miss hearing things, purposefully or through inattention, and improving the ability to listen is beneficial. As an example, increasing listening capability with an assistive listening device (a small electronic device that functions like a microphone) allowed otherwise healthy children with reading deficiencies to become better readers. Processing by their brains was changed, and the positive effects continued after the children's teacher no longer used the assistive listening device.

While AVT is directed at those with hearing loss, everyone can be a better listener, which can be achieved through listening to music. Musicians perceive more auditorily than nonmusicians. Dr. Nina Kraus tested musicians and nonmusicians on the ability to interpret simple sentences in a background of noise. The participants all had the same ability to hear, as shown with standard hearing tests. Despite identical hearing, the musicians showed a superior ability to correctly understand the spoken sentences.

Musicians are also better able to respond to specific sounds, in terms of quickness, accuracy, and focus. Dr. Kraus and colleagues tested this ability by asking musicians and nonmusicians to click a button when hearing a particular sound but not others. Musical ability has also been shown to train the brain to connect sound to meaning (notes to melody) over and over again. This kind of brain training aids neural processing of sound, much as exercising one's heart and legs by running changes the physical ability to handle long distances; exercising and training the brain using sounds improves one's ability to listen and respond. Music improves your listening ability and helps grow your language and reading skills.

In addition to music, using skills from improvisation (improv) can improve listening and communication. In improv, a theater technique, one listens and adds

MUSIC AND AUDITORY PERCEPTION

Musicians have courses in ear training that expand their ability to listen. They learn to distinguish different instruments, play a song that is heard just once, and communicate musical patterns in detail. Being able to describe music is analogous to having the words to portray a visual image. Visually, you can talk about color, shape, and size; you could say there is a red square that is larger than a yellow triangle. Those familiar with musical elements can accurately express the space between notes (interval), pitch (high vs. low sounds), timbre ("color" of sound), amplitude (loudness), and tempo (rate). Musicians are more able to define and hear these elements compared to nonmusicians.

Ear training is likely a key factor in the different listening skills of musicians and nonmusicians, and ear training impacts more than just musical ability. Musicians are better able to distinguish emotion in vocal tone than non-musicians. Musical training also helps people to hear better in noise and has been linked to gains in language skills. Anyone can capitalize on these listening benefits by learning to play an instrument.

on to what one has heard. Improv translates well to practicing listening – there is a measurable goal (one hundred percent of the time, say, *Yes, and...*) and lots of practice to learn from failing and success. With practice in improv, one learns to counter spontaneously and confidently in a positive manner, to affirm and build on whatever has come before, and such responses can become habit. Ultimately, whether through AVT, specialized equipment, music, or improv, thinking about listening and practicing listening helps us improve.

FOR ME: AUDITORY PERCEPTION

Teaching my son to listen expanded my world in ways I never thought imaginable. Continuously monitoring my son's listening ability using System 2 processing created my own System 1 listening habit. The four-year experience of growing my son's spoken language to a chronological age-matched level was full of challenges, but we were completely invested in targeting listening as an ability, setting measurable goals, and persevering through failing. We grew not only my son's listening ability during this time period but also my own ability to listen, to teach, to have patience, to learn, and use the techniques needed for each day or week or month. In training myself to listen to my son's articulations, I developed a listening habit around my son. It dawned on me that I might extend this habit to my doctoring relationships. I could listen better to my patients, which would help me gather more data for diagnosis and design a plan of treatment. I could be a better educator by listening more to the students and residents I was teaching. Instead of taking listening for granted in other relationships, *What would happen if I used a listening habit?*

DOCTOR-PATIENT CONNECTION: A LISTENING HABIT IS A SKILL

Like visual perception, "fast" (System 1) auditory processing is often taken for granted, unless one is deaf or hard of hearing. Most of us have experienced, however, difficulty hearing in noisy environments like a party or a concert. If you are invested in hearing at those times, you automatically listen differently. You may position yourself to hear optimally, leaning toward the other person or tilting your ear close to their mouth. You may consciously or subconsciously read lips. You may ask that the other person repeat what was said, use System 2 processing to double-check what you are hearing, or ask to move the conversation to someplace quieter. All of these accommodations represent intelligent use of perception. When needed, you can focus on your auditory perception – you can "turn the volume up".

KEY TAKEAWAY

While you can effortfully listen better in certain situations, those with typical hearing cannot actually turn the ears off. Loud, intermittent noise can and will be disturbing. Aside from disruptive sounds, sounds with particular meaning (e.g. your name) will grab your attention more readily. Auditory perception is ongoing, even during sleep; you cannot *not* hear, and in that sense, your ability is fixed. Some abilities are static. Had cochlear implants not worked for my son, in terms of giving him access to sound, there was no other current way to generate sound for him. His ability to hear sound through his ears would not be something that I could increase. Not everything can be changed. But even if my son didn't have access to sound, learning a different way to communicate

EVELYN GLENNIE: TEACHING THE WORLD TO LISTEN

Dame Evelyn Glennie is the world's first solo percussionist; she has recorded numerous albums and is widely recognized for her music. In 2015, she won the Polar Music Prize, the musical equivalent of the Nobel prize. Her mission is to Teach the World to Listen. And although she does not emphasize the fact, she is profoundly deaf.

Dame Glennie's focus is her music, but she recognizes that the spotlight is often on her deafness. Starting at about age eight, she doggedly learned to compensate for progressively worsening hearing loss. Her wonderful teachers coached her to listen with her body as her listening ability with her ears deteriorated. Her bare feet in the studio heard the vibrations through her soles and toes. She discriminated pitch by where she heard sound all over her body, her feet, her neck, her chest as examples. She says, "Losing my hearing made me a better listener", using her entire body as a giant ear, expanding the concept of auditory perception.

"Life begins and ends with listening."
— Dame Evelyn Glennie

would always still have been an option. If you don't meet the goals you set, you can learn from failing, think outside the box, and modify your next set of measurable goals.

If you are not constrained by access to sound, you can become a better listener through increasing your auditory perception. If you are a physician, listening to what you hear is a first step to saying the right thing. Some of us are more visual, and some of us are more auditory. Just as for vision, trying one of the exercises at the end of this chapter (yourself or with your family or friends) can prove to you that you can change your auditory intelligence. Your listening ability can be grown. You can learn a listening habit.

"Listen
to understand
rather than
listen
to respond."
— Barack Obama,
Former President of the USA

PRACTICAL APPLICATIONS:
A LISTENING HABIT

Play an instrument (learn to play if you don't know how) to grow your listening ability.

Reading aloud for 20 minutes a day is cumulative, and approximates to a staggering 1,800,000 words/year. *Close to 2 million words!* In contrast, reading for just five minutes a day translates to only 282,000 words/year.

Next time you are having a (difficult) conversation, aim for three *yeses* - repeat three things that were said and ask for a "yes, no" regarding if you have understood correctly.

"Listening is the backbone
to every aspect of our lives.
The challenges we face
in business and our domestic lives
can usually be overcome
with better listening skills."
—Dame Evelyn Glennie, Solo Percussionist, Three-
time Grammy Award Winner, and Winner of the
Polar Music Prize

FURTHER READING

176 Assistive listening device...Tallal P. Improving neural response to sound improves reading. *PNAS* 2012;109:16406-16407. AND Hornickel J, et al. Assistive listening devices drive neuroplasticity in children with dyslexia. *PNAS* 2012;109:16731-16736.

176 Musicians perceive more... Slater J, et al. Music training improves speech-in-noise perception: longitudinal evidence from a community-based music program. *Behav Brain Res* 2015;291:244-252.

177 Music improves your listening ability...Portas CM, Krakow K, Allen P, Josephs O, Armony JL, Frith CD. Auditory processing across the sleep-wake cycle: simultaneous EEG and fMRI monitoring in humans. *Neuron* 2000;28:991–999. AND Kraus N, et al. Music training for the development of auditory skills. *Nat Rev Neurosci* 2010;11:599-605. AND Kraus N, et al. Emergence of biological markers of musicianship with school-based music instruction. *Ann NY Acad Sci* 2015;1337:163-169.

178 Musicians are better able to distinguish emotion...Strait DL, et al. Musical experience and neural efficiency: Effects of training on subcortical processing of vocal expressions of emotion. *Eur J Neurosci* 2009;29:661-668.

178 Using skills from improvisation...Shochet R, et al. 'Thinking on my feet': An improvisation course to enhance students' confidence and responsiveness in the medical interview. *Educ for Primary Care* 2013;24:119-124.

182 Losing my hearing made me a better listener...
https://www.polarmusicprize.org/laureates/
evelyn-glennie/press-material

8 AUDITORY DATA FOR OPTIMIZING HEALTHCARE INTERACTIONS

"The quieter you become, the more you are able to hear."
—Rumi, Persian Poet

After my son's relatively late diagnosis of auditory neuropathy at age two, he had surgery for bilateral cochlear implantation. This was followed by many appointments, particularly with our auditory verbal therapist who was giving us the tools for my son to reach age-matched speech and language. During the first year, progress was a turtle, and our therapist told me to think of my son like an infant who isn't yet one year old. Language is being absorbed, but most babies don't say their first word until around age one. Of course, one of the difficulties with this is that my son was already over two years of age, not somewhere below age one, and most toddlers going through the terrible twos have a lot more language than my son. Imagine how frustrating it is to not be able to communicate your needs!

Prior to the surgery, doctors had predicted that cochlear implantation might not create enough access to sound, in which case speech and spoken language development would remain very difficult. This prognostication combined with our slow progress in the initial year prolonged my concern about my son's ultimate ability to develop spoken language the first two years (and more) post-surgery. Meanwhile, there were incremental gains that gave me hope that we would eventually win the race.

Once, as my son and I walked with our auditory verbal therapist down a hallway before a therapy session, we passed a beach scene posted on the wall, made out of construction paper. There were different colored buckets and sand shovels and kids playing.

The buckets and shovels reminded me that my son had pointed at a couple of objects in the past week, naming the colors, "blue", "red", and "yellow." I shared this information with our therapist as we went by, happy that he was saying more words.

Our therapist said bluntly, *Colors will get you nowhere in life*. I was walking slightly behind her, with my son next to me, and she didn't register my shock and dismay.

I regretted mentioning colors at all, wishing that I had kept my joy to myself.

SUBOPTIMAL COMMUNICATION

Our auditory verbal therapist cared greatly for my son, and I appreciated that her focus on his listening and language skills was unparalleled and uncompromising. Her ability as an auditory verbal therapist, I realized over time, was immense, and I was lucky to be learning from her. In terms of empathizing with me, I would say that she almost always did, and the story about the colors is unfair because it is a rare example of us disconnecting.

I will admit, though, that this brief conversation was enough to make me briefly consider transferring my son's care to someone else. Her response to my comment about colors hurt me, and the pain mattered, in the moment, more than her expertise. Luckily, I was scheduled to speak to the Director of the center soon thereafter, and during our talk, it came up that the families that stayed with our current therapist had the best outcomes for speech and language. With the lens of time, I am glad that I put my feelings aside and chose to stay with our therapist, who I knew cared greatly for us. I also wish that, at that time, I wouldn't have had to think about making that choice.

No one is perfect, and no relationship is going to be perfect. You try, you fight the battles that are essential, and you try again when you fail. I do this as a doctor, and I do this as the mother of a patient, and really, in all of my important relationships. And all of this applies to listening – I listen, I don't always interpret correctly, and I try again – both as a doctor and on the patient side and in other key relationships. Knowledge of auditory data, how it is processed, and ways to generate connection are all essential when we listen to create interpersonal connection.

YOUR LISTENING BANDWIDTH

The amount of information that the brain can consciously process at one moment can be estimated at about 100 units. You can think of this number as your bandwidth. When you are listening to one person speak, you are using about 60 units of that neural processing ability. The numbers explain why you are incapable of listening well to 2 different people at the same time – your brain does not have the bandwidth. You must consciously choose which person to listen to or lose parts of both messages. Some may feel they can listen to more than one person at the same time, in which case they are often only listening for particular content (and missing the rest). Everyone's listening bandwidth is limited by the human brain.

Considering this data from a different perspective, when one person is speaking, you have about 40 units of neural processing to spare. You may find your mind wandering, finding ways to use your extra processing ability, to your detriment, as you can miss crucial verbal messages. Certain phrases that do not have high priority content may lead to increased distraction. Such phrases are used more often by women than men and generally should be avoided if possible, particularly when they signify self-doubt. Examples include, "This is just me, but…" or "I'm sorry, but…" (when you are not actually apologizing for anything). Deleting these phrases helps listeners stay focused on your message, particularly if part of your message is dependent on communicating with authority, expertise, and confidence.

SPEECH NUTS AND BOLTS

There are important characteristics of speech, and working with a linguist has been shown to improve doctor-patient communication. Three things that are more accessible and easily observable include word choice, speed, and energy (see **Appendix** for a list of linguistic aspects communication). Overly complex language and ideas are not accessible to people. Simplified ideas and words present better. If doctors speak in "medicalese," patients are not as likely to understand compared to if doctors do their best to translate medical concepts into everyday language or terms that are accessible to patients. Doctors may use medicalese because that is their comfort zone, or medicalese may just be a consequence of not having thought out what explanation might make the most sense to a patient. In essence, using medicalese may also be habit – doctors become used to speaking about medical diagnoses in medical terms, over long and arduous years of training, and there is not necessarily the same degree of training in how best to communicate with patients.

In addition to word choice, speed is also important in communication – think of someone who talks excessively fast or extremely slowly. Language analysts can put a number on ideal speed, and a range of 100-200 words/minute is best. That's two to three words for every second – remember back to elementary school and think about the time it takes to say, "One Mississippi." A more rapid pace indicates passion, urgency, excitement, or strong emotion; a slower pace suggests importance or seriousness, sadness, or confusion. The tempo of your speech matters, and slower is usually better. Faster speech comes across as demanding or aggressive, while measured speech is perceived much more positively.

Gender and cultural differences also affect pace and speed. Especially in a relatively short patient visit, doctors may feel obliged to present things quickly, in order to cover everything necessary. But talking too fast for comprehension is not beneficial to the patient. Especially for key messages, it is important to speak at a slower pace.

In optimal communication, energy complements word choice and speed. Energy, on a basic level, is related to tone and volume. Imagine listening to someone who seems bored by their own words or conversely is bouncing off the walls. Neither situation is ideal. An appropriate amount of energy will aid comprehension in any conversation.

Adding on to word choice, speed, and energy, the concept of priming is useful. In healthcare interactions, when giving or receiving results, the patient might first ask, "Is it good news or bad news?" The question relates to priming, preparing oneself for what is to come. Before an important one-on-one conversation or speech in front of an audience, you need to choose priming words to increase effectiveness. These words are specially selected to emphasize how you want the listener to feel – a form of presetting the emotional state of the listener in real time, actively creating a particular bias for the listener. A concrete example is saying, "I have news" versus "I have exciting news" versus "I have disastrous news". In the first instance, you are not primed to feel anything. In the second, you expect something good, while the third statement causes you to brace yourself for an unpleasant revelation. Priming is also achieved by intonation – think of creating suspense with lowering the register of your voice as you say, "I have news." Priming sets the tone.

When you think about the message that you want to give someone, the last word will linger the most; you can be mindful of the last word you say in a sentence as well as the last word you say in an answer that you give. There is potentially a big difference between, "You have cancer" versus "You have cancer, and let's talk" for the listener. With the first, they may only hear and remember cancer. With the second, the patient can hopefully feel that they are not alone and together with the doctor, things can be discussed. Words and order matter, and in an unrehearsed conversation, messages can be easily lost or misinterpreted.

Something else to consider is that when you are speaking with authority, you may not convey emotions properly. Specifically naming your feelings is effective and helpful to the listener. For example, "I am saddened to give you this news." Naming the emotion can help drive the conversation forward with control and empathy.

Mirroring, framing, and humanizing statistics are three other linguistic aspects to be aware of. In mirroring, you repeat or rephrase some of the words or language of another person (or even your own prior statements), helping to reinforce a given message in order to aid retention of information and to validate the contribution of others. In framing, the same issue can be brought to light in different ways, just as in visual perception, the same shape can be perceived differently depending on context. Finally, relatable statistics, when spoken aloud, are also very effective at convincing people that they should continue listening. Ideally, statistics are put into humanized terms, in context, so that the numbers mean something and can be pictured in the mind's eye. For example, by February, 2021, the COVID-19 pandemic had killed more than 500,000 individuals in the United States. This death toll is more easily pictured in one's mind eye with these statistics: the death toll is greater than the number of Americans killed in both World War I and II, and 500,000 is about equal to the population of Atlanta, Georgia.

If you are data driven, you can explore speech even further, delving into the nuts and bolts of structure and technique. Speech itself can be quantified in different skill areas (see **Appendix** for a list of skill areas of speech) through linguistic analysis. Such analysis is performed by artificial intelligence as well as trained human evaluation (see **Appendix** for a sample linguistic report). With effort, each skill area can be improved; a communication coach can help.

TONE OF VOICE NUTS AND BOLTS

Emotion researchers have reported that there are at least five universal emotions that are recognized across cultures through corresponding facial cues and body maps. Universal emotions (see **Chapter 10**) are recognized by most emotion researchers, but not all. Emotions that have been identified similarly in different cultures include anger, disgust, fear, joy, and sadness. These five so-called "universal emotions" have also been shown to be encoded in tone of voice, termed vocal prosody, even when you use nonsense words or a foreign language. Interestingly, you can recognize fear most quickly (in about half a second), anger (in about three-quarters of a second), and happiness most slowly (which takes about one second). While this recognition time is slower than visual analysis of facial emotion, research has shown that you are able to detect emotion better when listening to vocal tone alone compared to a multi-sense situation like looking at a facial expression and listening to vocal tone. Vocal prosody has powerful nuance.

METAPERCEPTION IN LISTENING

You tend to take listening for granted if you have typical hearing, but most (this includes both medical professionals and patients) have never been taught how to actively listen in a relationship. Active listening involves not only speech but also body language, facial expression, and attentive silence. You must remember to hear the words spoken without getting overly distracted by your own thoughts. You should pay attention to body language, facial expression, tone of voice and other emotional information, but you also must not let that information overwhelm you before you even begin to process the actual words you hear.

According to Dr. Albert Mehrabian, like vs. dislike is transmitted largely by tone of voice and facial expression rather than speech. Additionally, going back to your brain's bandwidth, while average speech is about 125 words/minute, your thoughts run at a much higher pace. Because of this extra capacity of your brain, when you listen, you often begin to think of something else, especially if you are triggered in some way. Your thoughts can distract you from the speaker, and you may miss large chunks of data. Listening is not easy.

To strengthen healthcare relationships, you need to focus on listening and observing the words and body language of a patient. It is not necessarily effective to tell yourself, "Pay attention!" There are set actions that you can take to remain focused on the words you hear. Using your extra bandwidth, you can visually observe body language and facial expressions, compare your impressions with the words you are hearing, and assess for any discrepancies. If there is any incongruence, you can listen even more carefully to the words to detect what you might be missing. You can think about your existing emotional state as well as the speaker's and consider any bias that may be present; you should ask yourself if you or the speaker is mistaken in any judgments or conclusions (see **Chapter 3**). You can review periodically what has been said and weigh the validity of what is being said with what is known. Using the words that are heard, you can try to predict and interpret the speaker's ultimate idea or point. Being aware of conversational context will improve your ability to listen to speech.

KEY TAKEAWAY

With medical experience and proficiency as the solid base of a medical encounter, genuine listening without judgment or avoiding patient concerns strengthens healthcare relationships. Doctors should ask patients to rephrase what they have heard in their own words. Even if not asked, patients should repeat what they think they have heard, to make sure the interpretation is correct. Listening is important; double checking your listening will improve it.

CREATING A LISTENING HABIT FOR DOCTOR-PATIENT CONNECTION

DOCTOR

Start with the chief complaint, and habitually tag on, "Is there anything else you want addressed today?" This should help ensure the patient's needs and concerns are addressed.

Ask patients to "teach back" important healthcare concepts from the visit – to tell you, in their own words, what you have explained.

PATIENT

Make sure you listen for when your doctor asks what you want to cover in the visit. If your doctor doesn't ask in the first several minutes, make the opportunity to ask early on in the visit, "Would it be possible to make sure to cover ___ today?" If the physical examination has already started and you haven't had the chance to ask yet, it's okay to alert your doctor. Assuredly, it is best to let your doctor know as soon as possible what your goals for the visit are.

PRACTICAL APPLICATIONS: LISTENING

Read an internet article aloud, recording yourself. Try to vary the pace of your speech. Listen to your recording and assess any differences between your faster and slower speech. Bonus: paste the article into Microsoft Word or another program to do a word count in order to calculate out your words/minute.

The next time you are listening to someone, count how many times a minute you are able to mentally note the main points.

Monitor yourself next time you are listening to someone else speak. How many times does your mind wander? Or, for what percentage of the time does your mind wander while you are listening?

Next time you are listening to someone, try to a) notice body language and facial expressions, b) notice any incongruence, c) predict the main idea/ point, d) monitor any judgments you are making and test their validity by listening carefully to the words.

Role play with a friend or family member. Talk about a healthcare issue. Think about the words and the vocal tone used.

LANGUAGE AS A BARRIER IN HEALTHCARE INTERACTIONS

The importance of listening is evident in literature that shows significant barriers to healthcare that are created by differences in language or other ethnic/cultural considerations. Individuals who use signed language (see **Chapter 6**), for example, may not understand what they are being told by doctors in up to half of visits. Interpreters are not always readily available, exacerbating the problem.

All patients who use a different language than the local healthcare system's (e.g. English in the United States) benefit from translation services. Language can be difficult to separate from culture, and it has also been shown that patients who use a different language than the local one may also have cultural differences that create further miscommunication in healthcare interactions. Ideally, use of translators and cultural awareness will help decrease such disparities.

FURTHER READING

191 The amount of information that the brain can consciously process...Csikszentmihalyi M. *Flow: The Psychology of Optimal Experience*. New York: Harper Perennial Modern Classics, 1991.

191 About 60 units...Ibid.

192 Shown to improve doctor-patient communication...Wild D, Nawaz H, Ullah S, Via C, Vance W, Petraro P. Teaching residents to put patients first: Creation and evaluation of a comprehensive curriculum in patient-centered communication. *BMC Med Educ* 2018;18:266-274.

192 Word choice, speed, and energy...RoterDL, Frankel RM, Sluyter D. The expression of emotion through nonverbal behavior in medical visits. *J Gen Intern Med* 2006;21:S28-S34. AND William Vance, PhD. Lecture on Charisma, Yale Statement Makers, February, 2018.

192 If doctors speak in "medicalese"...Tate P, Frame F. *The Doctor's Communication Handbook*, 8th edition. Boca Raton: CRC Press, 2019; 1-142.

193 Not necessarily the same degree of training in how best to communicate with patients... Balakrishnan VS. In Shock: a book about compassion in the emergency department. *The Lancet Respiratory Medicine* 2018;6:92-93.

193 100-200 words/minute...William Vance, PhD. Personal communication, February, 2018.

194 The concept of priming is useful...Elgendi M, et al. Subliminal priming – State of the art and future perspectives. *Behav Sci (Basel)* 2018;8:54.

AND William Vance, PhD. Lecture on Charisma, Yale Statement Makers, February, 2018.

195 The last word will linger…William Vance, PhD. Personal communication, February, 2018.

196 Naming the emotion can help…Caruso D and Salovey P. *The Emotionally Intelligent Manager.* San Francisco: Jossey-Bass, 2004. AND Mayer JD, et al. The ability model of emotional intelligence: *Principles and Updates. Emotion Review* 2016;8:294.

196 Mirroring, framing, and humanizing statistics… Carr EW, et al. When mirroring is both simple and "smart": How mimicry can be embodied, adaptive, and non-representational. *Front Hum Neurosci* 2014;8:505. AND William Vance, PhD. Personal communication, February, 2018.

197 About equal to the population of Atlanta, Georgia…Rattner NF. U.S. surpasses 500,000 Covid deaths after yearlong battle with pandemic. https//www.cnbc.com/2021/02/22/the-us-covid-19-deaht-toll-has-surpassed-500000. html. Published 2021. Updated Monday, Feb 22, 2021 5 pm EST.

197 Emotion researchers…Ekman P. *Emotions Revealed.* New York: Times Books, 2013.

197 Universal emotions…Ibid.

197 Five so-called "universal" emotions have also been shown to be encoded in tone of voice… Liebenthal E, et al. The language, tone and prosody of emotions: neural substrates and dynamics of spoken-word emotion perception. *Front Neurosci* 2016;doi.org/10.3389/fnins.2016.

00506.

198 Recognize fear...Rigoulot S, et al. Feeling backwards? How temporal order in speech affects the time course of vocal emotion recognition. *Frontiers in Psychology* 2013;4;117.

198 Detect emotion better when listening to vocal tone...Kraus MW. Voice-only communication enhances empathic accuracy. *American Psychologist* 2017;72:644-654. AND Liebenthal E, et al. The language, tone and prosody of emotions: neural substrates and dynamics of spoken-word emotion perception. *Front Neurosci* 2016;doi.org/10.3389/fnins.2016.00506. AND Roter DL, Frankel RM, Sluyter D. The expression of emotion through nonverbal behavior in medical visits. *J Gen Intern Med* 2006;21:S28-S34. AND Riess H, Kraft-Todd G. E.M.P.A.T.H.Y.: A tool to enhance nonverbal communication between clinicians and their patients. *Acad Med* 2014;89:1108–1112.

199 Like vs. dislike is transmitted...Mehrabian A, Wiener M. Decoding of inconsistent communications. *J of Personality and Social Psychology* 1967;6:109-114. AND Mehrabian A, Ferris SR. Inference of attitudes from nonverbal communication in two channels. *J of Consulting Psychology* 1967;31:248-252.

199 Average speech is about 125 words/minute... Nichols RG and Stevens LA. Listening to people. https://hbr.org/1957/09/listening-to-people

203 LANGUAGE AS A BARRIER...

Al Shamsi H, Almutairi AG, Al Mashrafi S, Al Kalbani T. Implications of Language Barriers for Healthcare: A Systematic Review. *Oman Med J* 2020;35:e122.

Singleton K, Krause EM. Understanding cultural and linguistic barriers to health literacy. *Ky Nurse* 2010;58:4, 6-9.

9 EMOTION PERCEPTION: FORM A HABIT OF EMOTIONAL LOGIC BY THINKING ABOUT WHAT YOU FEEL, FAST AND SLOW

"Not the ones speaking the same language but the ones sharing the same feeling understand each other."
— Rumi, Persian Poet

I love what I do, but I had never intended to become a dermatologist.

I always had the preconceived notion that I would practice general medicine, become an "internist"; today referred to more commonly as a "primary care physician" or "non-special-ist". Internal medicine is MEDICINE, everything, all parts of the body, the interaction of beating hearts, breathing lungs, cleansing kidneys. I imagined my-self exploring the secrets of the human body, under-standing health and disease on a global level yet also in intimate, careful detail with healing being the holy grail. I didn't even consider being another type of doctor, and dermatology, a relatively small specialty that focuses on skin, hair, and nails, was not even on my radar.

During a critical training period in internal medicine as a third-year medical student, a cardiology fellow verbally abused me, her viciousness pelting daggers through the phone, her words accusing me of causing patient harm because he hadn't yet gotten a crucial procedure for his heart. This type of verbal abuse was apparently a pattern of the fellow's, but she was in rare form, shaming me and cursing at me as time seemingly stood still.

That day was the low point of medical school for me, the nadir of active clinical rotations during which there was a lot of real-time interaction with the messy actions and reactions of patients, other students, and physicians. None of the rotations had been easy or familiar to me, and unlike the majority of my classmates, I had a lot of nostalgia for the first two years of medical school, which had been abstract, tidy book-learning.

My ears still ringing, I immediately pushed the patient on his hospital bed to his procedure (the VA hospital had very little ancillary help), and then I left relatively early in the afternoon because my team had been "on call" (staying overnight) the night before. The sun was shining as I walked home, but the warm light was unable to dispel my dark mood and a subsequent hours-long storm of tears. Writing this story on paper, dredging up this memory, I still feel a bit ashamed of myself. I want to tell my younger self to buck up, move on, and ignore people who shout at you for no reason.

But the reality is that I just cried. And two of my friends did tell me (one more nicely than the other) that I was basically being a baby and I needed to function like an adult, like the doctor I was soon to become when I graduated with a medical degree. I should show them that I wasn't weak. I did return to work, early the next morning, at our regular time.

And that day the cardiology fellow found me and apologized to me for crossing the line. She was sincere in her remorse. The chief of internal medicine (the head of the entire service) called me into his sun-filled office the same day. He apologized as well for the cardiology fellow's actions; he was benevolently interested in me and my goals. He encouraged me, telling me that the team had told him that I was doing a great job. (The patient that I supposedly was killing was recovering well, as were all my patients.)

I had inadvertently proved my value, and no one at my sub-internship knew about my lengthy emotional breakdown of the previous day. I was viewed as a strong team member who had not complained despite ample reason. I now had a mentor to champion me, a respected internist and cardiologist who was strongly supportive of me and ready to back me in getting an excellent internal medicine spot for residency.

But I no longer wanted to be a doctor.

The loss of desire was inexplicable to me, but I made no attempt at that time to parse out reasons. Once my sub-internship was over, my attitude had not changed. I seriously considered quitting medical school, as internal medicine had been my goal. Truthfully, the only thing that stopped me was that I had no other skills. Certainly not ones related to emotional intelligence.

Almost two decades later, I began to process all my reactions more consciously, reviewing what had happened, analyzing my feelings, attaching emotion names to my experience. Instead of just crying (which actually can be an effective strategy when used properly), I began to think about my tears and loss of a life-long goal. At the time, I probably would have said that I was sad, had someone asked me to name an emotion. Looking back, I can see there was latent fear, which I didn't name then, that the cardiology fellow was right. Such analytical processing of my experience is what emotional intelligence is about – naming, managing, and using emotions deliberately rather than allowing them to inappropriately drown, distort, or determine what happens next. My tears made me feel powerless and impotent. Had I named my emotion as fear then, perhaps I would have been able to channel that into defending myself and protecting my goals, rather than running away.

My tears were like a tidal wave that submerged me. I didn't know how to interpret my ambiguous emotions effectively, and I had no idea how to manage them. The experience was a tipping point for me, and instead of confronting how overwhelming a critical sub-internship can be, I mentally jumped ship. I considered not finishing medical school. Despite the apologies that were given the following day, my change-of-heart persisted. I didn't become an internal medicine doctor because of this one experience. Applying the skills of emotional intelligence might have been able to alter that outcome.

EMOTIONAL INTELLIGENCE

Emotional intelligence was popularized by Daniel Goleman, PhD as predicting greater success for individuals compared to the traditional intelligence quotient. While the concept of emotional intelligence has taken on many different meanings, the focus here is on the skill of emotional intelligence as put forth by Drs. Peter Salovey and David Caruso. In *The Emotionally Intelligent Manager*, Drs. David Caruso and Peter Salovey outline a simple 4-step process for using emotional intelligence effectively. These skills are important for building strong relationships. Four steps help you to be "both effective *and* compassionate". These steps include reading people's emotions (identifying emotions), matching the emotions to the task (using emotions), understanding the causes of the emotions and predicting the emotional future (understanding emotions), and staying open to the data conveyed by the emotions (managing emotions). Using emotional intelligence prevents you from assuming that emotions are bad and takes you into a space where emotions can be helpful; this transition is important because labeling emotions correctly actually helps you be more effective. Specific to doctors, emotional intelligence has been linked to improved clinical performance and medical interviewing as well as decreased burnout in the healthcare setting.

Dr. Caruso has simplified the model of emotional intelligence with a simple "blueprint" – Map, match, ascribe meaning to move emotions (see **Appendix**). Map refers to "mapping" basic elements of your emotions, matching to correlating emotions (yours and others) to the problem at hand; the last two are related, using the meaning and trajectory of emotions to move emotions on that map to attain a goal. Just as you perceive your surrounding environment, visual and auditory, to help guide your thinking and planning, emotions should also be treated as information to channel next steps. Emotional logic and logical emotions are not oxymorons. Emotions are a useful conduit to optimize your effectiveness.

To better understand the skill of emotional intelligence, a basic understanding of cognition is useful. Metacognition is thinking about how you think, and Nobel prize-winning Dr. Daniel Kahneman created constructs for two major thinking patterns – fast thinking and slow thinking – dubbed System 1 and System 2 thinking. System 1, fast thinking, is gut reaction, habit, expert thinking. System 2, slow thinking, is more conscious and controlled. Thinking carefully about our emotions is a form of metacognition, and just as with thinking, you have "fast" and "slow" emotion perception. Emotions are not separate from cognition, and just like System 1 and System 2, emotions and emotional intelligence are semantic constructs that aid emotion metaperception (see **Appendix**).

Emotional intelligence is critical for doctors and patients. Patients and doctors have emotions (System 1, "fast emotions"), whether those emotions are picked up on or not. Awareness of those relatively automatic emotions (System 2, "slow" analysis of feelings) prevents physician burnout and leads to increased doctor and patient satisfaction. Unfortunately, the Dunning-Kruger effect (rating your level of competence higher than one's true competence, particularly when unskilled; see **Introduction**) often comes into play, and self-rated emotional intelligence does not accurately predict positive patient-doctor interactions. This means if you believe you are highly emotionally intelligent you may not be. Of even greater importance, other research indicates most people overestimate their level of emotional intelligence, and the more a person overestimates their emotional intelligence, the less interested he/she is in developing these skills.

What does this mean for doctor-patient communication? Patients, already in a somewhat compromised position, may feel uncomfortable expressing emotion. And, as noted above, doctors' emotional intelligence may be lower than they think, so there is a good chance the doctor is not picking up on patients' concerns or fears. A doctor asks, "Is everything okay?", accepts the patient's, "Umm, sure," and does not sense the patient's anxiety which signals that *No, everything is definitely not okay*. There can be a loss of an important source of information.

Doctors and patients may think that it is more intelligent to suppress emotion and focus on another important task at hand – proper medical diagnosis and treatment. Both doctors and patients may consider healthcare visits to be more successful each time both parties are able to "keep it together" during the doctor-patient interaction by concealing any emotions. Before we accept this type of supreme control as ideal, consider the work of Stanford psychologist James Gross on suppressing emotion. Gross and colleagues found that suppressing your emotion display requires cognitive resources and consequently results in recalling less information. Think about your own experience for a moment where someone said something which angered you. Rather than blurting out how you felt, you suppressed any expression of anger. In the next moment, you might realize you missed what the other person said and might need to ask, "I'm sorry; what did you say?" While it is not recommended that you impulsively act on your unexamined, or even examined, feelings, consider that suppression of emotion is not necessarily the best emotion management strategy. Interestingly, doctors who express more emotion, even nonverbally, are seen more positively by patients.

Labeling emotions is a good start to using emotional intelligence in doctor-patient interactions. This helps not only discrete doctor-patient interactions but also future ones, for the doctor, patient, and anyone else present. In particular, if trainees are involved, actively recognizing potential difficulties in handling emotions when caring for patients helps physician teachers provide better models of emotional intelligence for students. Unfortunately, the traditional curriculum in most medical schools generally has not taught such skills, particularly to more senior faculty members who trained in the past.

EMOTION ILLUSIONS

Just as there are optical and auditory illusions in which you see or hear something that is not there, emotion illusions exist. Emotion illusions are the opposite of emotional intelligence and generally steer you in the wrong direction. If you think of emotion illusions as analogous to optical illusions, an emotion illusion can be defined as the perception of an emotion that is not there, misperceiving what is there, or ignoring what is there. Such illusory emotions have been termed "recalcitrant emotions", or emotions that are out of sync with factual judgment. An important difference between a recalcitrant emotion and an optical illusion (see **Chapter 5**) is that the latter may not need to be managed so that you act appropriately. If you see 2 circles as being of different size when they are identical (see **Chapter 5**), this misperception does not necessarily cause any major negative consequence. Recalcitrant emotions often do lead to actions, and they may be irrational and illogical or the converse.

Being yelled at certainly will cause an emotion for most people, as it did for me during my sub-internship. I believe my illusory emotion was sadness, which could in part explain my loss of desire to become a doctor. Looking back, I think the stronger (but unrecognized) emotion was fear, and perhaps naming that emotion would have helped me manage the situation and my ultimate reaction differently and more effectively. The importance of considering emotion illusions rests in questioning whether your emotions are leading you appropriately. Particularly when you come to a fork in the road, emotional intelligence is useful.

HOW THIS APPLIES TO DOCTORS AND PATIENTS

While each of us is more or less emotional and aware of emotions, emotions have been shown to be crucial to proper decision-making, perception, and attention; emotional connection even enhances or inhibits memory. Individuals with neurological brain damage in targeted areas can retain high levels of intellectual function but decision-making can be highly impaired. Conversely, heightened awareness of emotions can also improve your decisions. Emotions are very much a part of intelligent decisions; even subliminal emotion can be influential, without conscious realization.

Using emotional intelligence, you can identify emotions (see **Chapter 10**), use them to guide your thinking through evaluating possible outcomes and ultimately synthesize that data into an optimal response. We all have variably strong emotions. But your ultimate interpretation and response are not uncontrollable. While babies are too young to manage their emotions, even toddlers can manage emotional reactions with the proper tools. Using emotions to the benefit of people is emotional intelligence.

FOR ME: EMOTIONS

Emotion awareness is not easy for me; my System 1, "fast" emotional logic is weak. Growing up, I never talked about feelings. In my family, there was not much communication, in general. We never even said, *I love you*. A lot was just supposed to be understood, a given, known without naming. And overall, as my sister says, I was a "happy camper". Coming from a happy place, I had an active imagination for overwrought melodrama; I wrote bad poetry, love songs, and even a romance novel where somehow the villain became the hero but was stuck with his original, heinous name of Delmond Snypof. According to my mother, she expected us to study hard and get good grades, and since we did, she didn't think it necessary to intrude. There was also a language and cultural barrier. My mother thought her English was poor, and our Korean wasn't that great. My father's English was and is excellent, but he was often working and absent from home life. Emotional intelligence was not part of my childhood, and it was not something I was taught in school.

My emotional intelligence journey started once I had two children, through auditory verbal therapy (see **Chapter 8**) and my daughter's school. When my daughter started kindergarten, her school brought up communicating to our kids about emotions. In auditory verbal therapy, we used deliberate language to talk about emotions. Learning about emotions (for the first time!) at home with my children was System 2, "slow" work, and it made me precipitously aware of how little emotional recognition I had up to that point in my own life. My lack of awareness suddenly seemed foolish; I slowly came to realize that treating my emotions as the unwelcome stepchild, relegated to the shadows, likely was making me less effective.

Particularly at work, but also at base, I tended

"The emotional brain responds to an event more quickly than the thinking brain."
— Daniel Goleman, Author of *Emotional Intelligence*

to think of emotions as an unprofessional weakness, and I am not alone in this thinking. Both positive and negative emotions have display rules at work, and while anger is a commonly experienced emotion in the workplace, and expressing anger is often viewed as a strength, many emotions are masked, even in the critical doctor-patient relationship and among physicians.

As I got better at recognizing and using emotions at home, I began to apply the skills of emotional intelligence at work. I still don't think that my own emotions, in all their glory, should be on full display at work, but it is important to be able to recognize emotions in myself, in patients, and others; validate those emotions; and treat them with logic.

DOCTOR-PATIENT CONNECTION: THE HABIT OF EMOTIONAL LOGIC IS A SKILL

Being able to identify the emotions engendered in yourself and others, by each other as well as the environment (e.g. art, music), is an art form that some are better at than others. As with any skill, like drawing or playing an instrument, naming and mapping emotions is something that you can get better at. You can learn to recognize the maelstrom of emotions swirling around you. You can channel your emotions logically and productively.

As you become more aware of emotions and their influence, you can use pleasant or "positive" emotions to brainstorm and use unpleasant or "negative" emotions to focus on details. Emotions, like colors, fall along a predictable continuum, with variation in intensity and different relationships. Familiarity with colors helps you to know that mixing red and blue make purple, pink can be considered a lighter shade of red, and opposing colors are opposites on a color wheel (e.g. red and green). Similar fluency with emotions allows you to recognize that initial frustration plus continued provocation can turn into anger; fear promotes anger; and sadness, fear, and anger can all counter happiness. Understanding and predicting these patterns is emotional intelligence.

"...the little emotions are the great captains of our lives and we obey them without realizing it."

— Vincent Van Gogh, Artist

CHANNELING BASIC EMOTIONS AND THEIR SPECTRUM

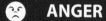 **ANGER**

When productive:
Gives you power and energy
Helps you correct injustice

Spectrum: Skepticism, irritation, frustration, indignation, jealousy, hurt, resentment, fury, rage

DISGUST

When productive:
Sets rules of acceptability
Helps you follow rules

Spectrum: Disapproval, distaste, objection, hesitancy, avoidance, loathing

FEAR

When productive:
Alerts you
Helps you recognize errors

Spectrum: Concern, worry, anxiety, insecurity, submissiveness, humiliation, overwhelm, panic, terror

HAPPINESS

When productive:
Inspires you
Helps you keep going

HAPPINESS, CONT.
Spectrum: Contentment, peace, confidence, pleasure, optimism, power, pride, happiness, playfulness, delight, elation

SADNESS
When productive:
Deals with loss
Helps you rely on others

Spectrum: Thoughtfulness, pensiveness, disappointment, boredom, loneliness, abandonment, desperation, apathy, emptiness, guilt, distress, shame, grief, misery*

The five "basic" emotions here are recognized and named more easily by young children and adults. In contrast, the spectrum listed below each basic emotion is different in terms of lexical complexity, level of associated energy, and positive or negative valence. Just as variations of the color red (e.g. crimson, rose, wine) are not perceived exactly the same way by all individuals, these emotional states may also be graded differently by others. The point of recognizing basic/universal emotions and those of different intensity lies in naming and managing these emotional states for your benefit.

Emotions are a construct and are "very likely perceptually categorized and experienced as a single unified percept, much like color, depth, and shape are experienced together in object perception". Just as the color red is seen via wavelengths of red light that are experienced as red, a given emotion is experienced from a "continuous stream of evolving affect and conceptual processing". Not only is red seen as a color, red can have other effects on the brain – red causes you to be more alert, appear more attractive, and have more success in sports. The perception of red around you affects behavior.

Similarly, in so-called emotional contagion, perceived emotions in your surroundings can affect your behavior. If someone else is happy, you are more likely to be happy. If someone else is angry, you pick up on that anger and feel that way yourself. It's important to note the more powerful the person, the more emotionally contagious they are, something to be aware of in doctor-patient interactions. When you sense these emotions, you are more likely to feel a certain way. Through emotional intelligence, you can channel this knowledge productively, neither being ruled by your emotions nor neglecting them.

KEY TAKEAWAY

For anyone who remains uncomfortable with emotions, discomfort may dissipate through knowing that research has shown that emotions follow logical patterns. Dr. Caruso suggests that, "People often do not trust their emotions and are told to disregard them. Good advice if the bad feeling is based on a mood or if you are lower on emotional intelligence because your analysis of the root cause will likely be wrong. Go with your gut [System 1, "fast" emotion] is terrible advice; go with your analyzed gut [System 2, "slow" emotion] is good advice." You may not be able to harness every emotion that you feel, but on a simplified level, you can control what you do with your emotions once you understand their inherent reliability.

Dr. Caruso uses the analogy of a jet for the power of emotions and channeling their power: For example, think of anger as jet fuel – it has raw energy and simply tossing a match at the fuel will cause an explosion; instead, with highly developed skills, engineers design, model, test, refine and harness the energy of that fuel with a sophisticated jet engine, and trained pilots at the controls learn to harness the power to achieve flight. Likewise, in the hands of many of us, anger and other emotions can be destructive or can be used constructively to create something positive. Both doctors and patients can develop their emotional intelligence skills through deliberate practice, thoughtfulness and modeling, and corrective feedback over a period of time.

"Reason without affect would be impotent, affect without reason would be blind."
— Silvan Tomkins, American Psychologist and Personality Theorist

PRACTICAL APPLICATIONS:
A HABIT OF EMOTIONAL LOGIC

Think about the following when you feel an emotion, three times a day for one week. (Adapted from Dr. Caruso.)

- How strong is this feeling?
- Is it unusual for me to feel this way?
- How might someone else feel in this situation?
- What was my background mood at the time?
- And the key question: How much of this feeling is due to my mood (background "noise") and how much of my feeling is due to an emotion (a "figure" or "event" superimposed on the background noise)?

Fill out a mood scale three times a day for two weeks.

Start an emotion diary and continue with it for three months.

Each interaction that you have, name one emotion, and consider how best to manage it.

EMOTION PERCEPTION: MUSIC

Music can engender emotions in listeners, and film scorers use this propensity to enhance movies. The presence or absence of music can emphasize certain scenes, and the same melody can provide continuity between scenes, much as the same visual background might do. Upbeat music often accompanies the introduction of a hero, while unnerving music introduces villains. Fast-paced, complex music enhances a chase scene, slow tempo music augments sadness, and sharp, piercing sounds heighten fear. Music is linked to emotion.

In everyday life, people also use music to regulate emotions. Sad songs can paradoxically induce pleasure, and they have also been shown to enhance empathy and emotional regulation. By listening to a sad song, the listener's mood can improve through the richness of the music, feeling empathy by appreciating the sadness induced through listening, and allowing time for self-reflection.

JOHN MCENROE

John McEnroe is an American tennis player with 77 singles and 78 doubles titles. He was named the ATP Player of the year and ITF World Champion in 1981, 1983, and 1984. He is a tennis legend, known for his tennis skills but also his emotional outbursts.

John McEnroe never held back his palpable anger, a tidal wave of ferocity expressed with his body language and speech. His face and body language were wildly expressive as he harangued referees. He would break tennis racquets. He would curse.

After retirement, he noted that he never tried to control his anger and channel it productively – his anger took over, was destructive, and could lead to a loss. He says of his opponents, "I'd start belittling them and then they'd start trying twice as hard and I'd lose…it would get in the way of my performance." Getting in your own way is something that you don't want; the energy of emotions should not shift your momentum in the wrong direction.

FURTHER READING

214 Emotional Intelligence was popularized...Goleman D. *Emotional Intelligence: Why It Can Matter More than IQ.* New York: Bantam Books, 1995.

214 Skill of emotional intelligence...Caruso D and Salovey P. *The Emotionally Intelligent Manager.* San Francisco: Jossey-Bass, 2004. AND Mayer JD, et al. The ability model of emotional intelligence: Principles and updates. *Emotion Review* 2016;8:294.

215 Emotional intelligence has been linked...Sattefield J, et al Emotional intelligence in internal medicine residents: Educational implications for clinical performance and burnout. *Ann Behav Sci Med Educ* 2009;14:65-58.

215 Dr. Caruso has simplified...Caruso DR, Rees LT. *A leader's guide to solving challenges with emotional intelligence.* Publishing Genius Press, 2018.

216 Dr. Daniel Kahneman created constructs...Kahneman D. *Thinking, Fast and Slow.* New York: Farrar, Straus and Giroux, 2011. p. 82.

217 "fast emotions"...Channouf A. Subliminal exposure to facial expressions of emotion and evaluative judgments of advertising messages. *Eur Rev Appl Psychol* 2000;50:19-23. AND Dimberg U, et al. Unconscious facial reactions to emotional facial expressions. *Psychol Sci* 2000;11:86-89.

217 The Dunning-Kruger effect...Kruger J et al. Unskilled and unaware of it: How difficulties in recognizing one's own incompetence lead to inflated self-assessments. *J Personal Soc Psychol*

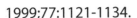

1999;77:1121-1134.

217 Other research indicates most people…Sheldon OJ, Dunning D, & Ames DR. Emotionally unskilled, unaware, and uninterested in learning more: Reactions to feedback about deficits in emotional intelligence. *Journal of Applied Psychology* 2014;99:125–137.

218 Consider the work of Stanford psychologist… Richards JM, Gross JJ. Emotion regulation and memory: The cognitive costs of keeping one's cool. *J Personality Soc Psychol* 2000;79:410-424.

219 Doctors who express more emotion, even nonverbally, are seen more positively…Roter DL, Frankel RM, Sluyter D. The expression of emotion through nonverbal behavior in medical visits. *J Gen Intern Med* 2006;21:S28-S34.

220 Recalcitrant emotions…Tappolet C. Chapter 11: Emotions, perceptions, and emotional illusions. In: Calabi C. (eds). *Perceptual illusions*. London: Palgrave Macmillan, 2012.

221 Emotions have been shown to be crucial to proper decision-making…Pourtois G, et al. Brain mechanisms for emotional influences on perception and attention: What is magic and what is not. *Biological Psychology* 2013;92:492-512. AND Bechara A, et al. Emotion, decision making and the orbitofrontal cortex. *Cerebral Cortex* 2000;10:295-307. AND Damasio AR. Fundamental feelings. *Nature* 2001;413:781.

221 Emotions are very much a part of intelligent decisions…Bechara A, Damasio H, Damasio AR. Role of the amygdala in decision-making. *Ann*

NY Acad Sci 2003;985:356-369. AND Bechara A, et al. Different contributions of the human amygdala and ventromedial prefrontal cortex to decision-making. *J Neurosci* 1999;19:5473-5481.

224   Both positive and negative emotions have display rules at work...Kramer MW, et al. Communication rules for the display of emotions in organizational settings. *Management Communication Quarterly* 2002;16:66-80.

224   Anger is a commonly experienced emotion... Miron-Spektor E, et al. The effects of anger in the workplace: When, where, and why observing anger enhances or hinders performance. *Research in Personnel and Human Resources Management* 2009;28:153-178.

225   E.g. art, music...Gatti E, et al. Emotional ratings and skin conductance response to visual, auditory and haptic stimuli. *Sci Data* 2018;5:180120. AND Cupchik G, et al. Viewing artworks: Contributions of cognitive control and perceptual facilitation to aesthetic experience. *Brain and Cognition* 2009;70:84-91. AND Barry A. Perceptual aesthetics: Transcendent emotion, neurological image. *Visual Communication Quarterly* 2006;13:134-151.

225   "positive" emotions...Fredrickson BL. The value of positive emotions. *American Scientist* 2003;91:330-335. AND Palfai TP, et al. The influence of depressed and elated mood on deductive and inductive reasoning. *Imagination, Cognition, and Personality* 1993;13:57-71.

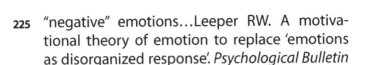

225 "negative" emotions...Leeper RW. A motivational theory of emotion to replace 'emotions as disorganized response'. *Psychological Bulletin* 1948;55:5-21.

225 Fear promotes anger...Zhan J, et al. The neural basis of fear promotes anger and sadness counteracts anger. *Neural Plasticity* 2018;doi.1155/2018/3479059.

225 Frustration plus continued provocation...Caruso D and Salovey P. *The Emotionally Intelligent Manager.* San Francisco: Jossey-Bass, 2004, pp. 19-20.

228 Very likely perceptually categorized...Barrett LF, et al. The experience of emotion. *Annu Rev Psychol* 2007;58:373-403.

228 Emotions are a construct...Barrett LF. The theory of constructed emotion: an active inference account of interoception and categorization. *Soc Cog Aff Neurosci* 2017;1-23.

228 Continuous stream of evolving affect...Ibid.

228 As a color, red...https://www.scientificamercan.com/article/how-the-color-red-influences-our-behavior/

228 So-called emotional contagion...Barsade SG. The ripple effect: emotional contagion and its influence on group behavior. *Administrative Science Quarterly* 2002;47:644-675.

229 Emotions follow logical patterns...Caruso DR, Rees LT. *A leader's guide to solving challenges with emotional intelligence.* Publishing Genius Press, 2018.

232 Music can engender emotion…Scherer KR. Which emotions can be induced by music? What are the underlying mechanisms? And how can we measure them? *J New Music Res* 2004;33:239-251.

232 Music is linked to emotion…https://www. epidemicsound.com/blog/music-and-emo-tion/ AND Taruffi L, et al. The paradox of mu-sic-evoked sadness: an online survey. *PLOS One*; doi.org/10.1371/journal.pone.0110490.

232 Music to regulate emotions…**Selected refer-ences:** Cook T, Ashlin RK, Welker KM. Music as an emotion regulation strategy: An examination of genres of music and their roles in emotion reg-ulation. *Psychol Music* 2017;47:144-154. AND Hides L, Dingle G, Quinn C, Stoyanov SR, Zelen-ko O, Tjondronegoro D, Johnson D, Cockshaw W, Kavanagh DJ. Efficacy and outcomes of a mu-sic-based emotion regulation mobile app in dis-tressed young people: Randomized controlled trial. *JMIR Mhealth Uhealth* 2019;7:e11482.

233 John McEnroe…https://theguardian.com/sport/ 2018/jul/08/john-mcenroe-mellowed-killer-in-stinct-wimbledon-bjorn-borg-roger-federer/

10 EMOTION DATA FOR OPTIMIZING HEALTHCARE INTERACTIONS

"Human behavior
flows
from three main
sources:
desire,
emotion,
and
knowledge."
—Plato,
Greek
Philosopher

Before I got married, my husband and I had two sessions of mandatory marriage counseling with our pastor. I hardly remember much of what we covered, but I distinctly recall one of the very first questions he asked us.

What do you like most about this person?

I immediately said, *He is a rock, stable, steady, reliable.*

My husband said, *She is very emotional, unlike me.*

You would think that we would have talked about these things, at some point, prior to being in marriage counseling. What is it that we like most about each other? Why are we truly choosing each other? Even now, I think love is hard to define, like many abstractions. While my husband is right, and I am quite emotional in the sense that I construct emotions quite readily, my instinctive understanding of those same emotions is relatively poor.

I also tend to think being emotional is negative, and I remember that as we drove away from our first counseling session, I asked my then fiancé, *Really? That's what you like most about me? That I'm emotional? Isn't that a bad thing?*

THE PROBLEM WITH EMOTIONS

My innate tendency toward being emotional is something that I have always considered to be a weakness. I have a bias against emotions, tending to think that they are unreliable, illogical, and unpredictable. I don't think I am alone in thinking this, and while sometimes emotions are unreliable, illogical, and unpredictable, even the most logic-based person has emotions.

I have come to slowly realize that emotions are data; they are useful. The more that I feel and am able to acknowledge my emotions, my life becomes fuller through channeling those emotions productively. Emotions should not be ignored.

Acceptance of the range of emotions I feel as a doctor and as the mother of a patient helps me function better in both roles. Being aware of how I feel and how that influences my interactions is invaluable. Thinking more about how my patients feel, and when I am on the other side, how my own doctors feel, changes the interaction, almost always in a positive direction. Being emotional and channeling it properly are useful.

EMOTION NUTS AND BOLTS

Emotions make you human, and we are all emotional. You vary in your expressivity and awareness of your own and others' emotions; more conscious awareness of emotions is emotional intelligence. Naming emotions is helpful as a first step in using your emotions effectively. Five basic (sometimes termed "universal") emotions (see also **Chapter 9**) – anger, disgust, fear, happiness, and sadness – have been recognized across cultures through corresponding facial cues and body maps. These five emotions are commonly expressed by both children and adults through body language, actions, and sometimes words (see **Appendix**).

Certain facial expressions correlate with particular basic emotions, and in general, such facial expressions are rapidly associated with a given emotion almost automatically and unconsciously. Smiling, which signifies happiness, generally leads to positive perceptions, including attractiveness, although the smile needs to be genuine, as assessed by involving the perioral muscles, but not too broad, as the latter reduces perceptions of competence. Just because someone's lips are shaped in a smile does not mean that the person is feeling happiness. Emotions are also expressed in the body, represented pictorially through body maps of where emotions localize. While you cannot see your own facial expression

---

*Joy and enjoyment can be considered synonyms for happiness. ~80% of researchers agree on these five basic/universal emotions.

RECOGNIZING BASIC EXPRESSIONS

Anger

Eyebrows low, eyes protruding and may be open wide, lips pressed together

Disgust

Nose wrinkled, eyebrows low, upper lip raised but relaxed; tongue may be sticking out

Fear

Eyebrows straight, raised; eyes wide open to show whites of eyes, mouth slightly open with lips stretched/tense

Happiness
(Enjoyment, Joy*)

Smiling: corners of mouth and cheeks raised, corners of eyes tightened/crinkled, teeth exposed

Sadness

Inner eyebrows raised, corners of mouth lowered, upper eyelids drooping

without a mirror, you can feel energy in your body, helping you name your emotions.

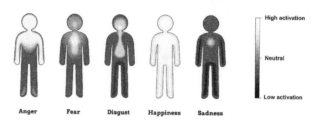

Colloquially, "emotion", "feeling", and "mood" are often used synonymously, but these terms are not synonymous to emotion researchers. (It is beyond the scope of this chapter and book, but on a more psychologically primitive and basic level, "core affect" is likely the better neurobiological term for what is thought of as "mood", "emotion", or "feeling" colloquially – core affect is the ever-present response of mind and body to different stimuli.) According to Dr. David Caruso, feelings are composed of both mood and emotion, and so, it is not always clear what your feelings are conveying, if anything. You can think of mood as the background, and an emotion

Body maps adapted from Volynets S, et al. Bodily maps of emotions are culturally universal. Emotion 2019;doi:10.1037/emo0000624.

is a figure that is overlaid on that background; the overall picture, the blend of mood and emotion, may or may not be clear or a reliable source of information. Visually, when you look at something, you automatically assign value – there is figure, and there is background. For hearing, when you listen to someone, you also assign value; there are the tone and words of the person's voice as well as background noise. You generally attend more to what you assign as a figure, but the background often influences everything around it. Your perception of what is seen, heard, and felt in a given instance is the combination of the background and the figure; reiterating this concept as applied to what we feel – mood is background, emotion is figure, and feelings are the blending of figure and ground.

Another way to help conceptualize feelings, mood, and emotion is to consider the physiologic expression of emotion, and your physical heart is a good example. You are generally not constantly, consciously aware of your beating heart, but the sensation is always there, just as some sort of mood is always present. You can sense a change sometimes – this would be an emotion overlaid on that mood –

your heart might start to race, either from excitement or fear or anger. That rapid heartbeat can happen somewhat automatically, without your consciously thinking about it, and you can sense it. The overall state of your heart (the feeling) is influenced by your baseline heart rate (mood) and any changes like acceleration (emotion). The baseline of your heart (the mood) needs to be managed to keep your heart healthy; you can do this through a proper diet and exercise. Examples of changes (emotions) overlaid on your baseline rate would include target heart rate during exercise, irregular heart beats, and effects on blood pressure. The data compared to baseline is important information that should be attended to.

Using these definitions of emotions, feelings, and moods helps separate emotions from what follows. Emotions come on quickly, are of relatively short duration, direct our attention, and ready us for action. Despite this automaticity, feelings are constructed, often given positive or negative attributes as you reflect on and process your emotions. If we think again to emotions as analogous to your heart rate, a rapid heart rate can be either helpful or troubling; the fast pumping of the heart helps a sprinter move faster while a too quick, irregular heartbeat can signify a medically significant heart issue. Similarly, emotions are often categorized as good or bad likely due to the sequelae of different emotions; sequelae may be relatively quick (e.g. a transient facial expression) or something that evolves more slowly over time (e.g. speaking loudly and forcefully in an argument). While emotions can be very intense, the actions that follow are what matters in relationships. You will be better able to leverage your emotions if you are able to recognize and label your emotions.

Five basic (or "universal") emotions, generally recognized across many cultures, have corresponding facial expressions that you "read" on others' faces, processing that information as quickly as 30 milliseconds. Such visual processing of facial expressions is an ability that can be changed. Emotions have nuance, and being able to label more accurately can help your interpretation. Gradation of different basic emotions can be appreciated through semantics (see **Chapter 9**). For example, anger runs on a spectrum from low-grade irritation or annoyance or frustration to extremes like fury or rage. Fear might range from a low-grade concern to outright terror.

Through first correctly labeling emotions, you have a much better chance at controlling your feelings, mood, and any response. Dr. Paul Ekman, who has authored many papers on emotions and facial expressions, has courses for *microexpression training.* You can actively learn, with practice, to consciously note subtle changes in facial patterns that correspond to different emotions.[1] In addition to facial patterns, there are vocalizations and body language that often correspond to a particular emotion. Body movements also transmit emotion, across different cultures, with the types of body movements being similar to the rate and rhythm of music that gives listeners the same feeling. While more recent research by Dr. Lisa Feldman Barrett suggests that emotion is constructed (rather than an innate neurobiologic reaction), the construction and understanding of emotion is still based on context, past learning, and experience. Thus, learning about emotion, facial expression, and body language can help you label emotions.

---

[1] Context is often important to correct interpretation of facial expressions.

METAPERCEPTION AND EMOTIONAL LOGIC

You can use logic to control your response to emotions using emotional intelligence. We all know that certain things "push our buttons". You can use so-called "affective forecasting" to predict emotions in yourself and others. Becoming aware of emotions, and learning to react in a different way is the process of self-control. Emotions are neither "bad" nor "good". You may think of anger as bad, because more often than not, you have seen negative actions result from anger, and you may have been taught to ignore or hide anger, but you are better off when you recognize it, feel it, and consciously control what you do next. The response to emotions is what leads to a bad or good outcome.

Accurately responding to your emotions is predicated on naming your emotions. If emotions are difficult to label, you can start in a relatively easy way by labeling the emotions of characters on TV or in books or in music itself, to neutralize the labeling of emotion. Another way to start would be to start with a mood meter or map; Dr. Caruso and colleagues have developed one. You can map your degree of "pleasantness" and "energy level" on such a map and in this way "look up" how best to label your emotional state.

Being aware of emotions is important as you generally are unable to fully cover up your emotions. Emotions are present, expressed, and interpreted by others, whether or not you are conscious of transmitting them. Your facial expressions show your emotions, and your emotions determine your facial expressions. Similarly, tone of voice and body language can convey emotion. Words themselves, which can be congruent or not with your body language and tone of voice, are also a component of emotions.

Emotions are an ingrained human construct, but you may not have emotional awareness. Lack of emotional awareness will lead to missing and misinterpreting emotional cues, including during healthcare interactions.

You can increase your emotion mindfulness by using contextual clues. As an example, we tend to be on the lookout for anger. Some argue that this sensitivity to anger is evolutionary, as anger can be considered a danger signal. Anger is often mismanaged, perhaps making us even more wary of it. We are particularly receptive to even subtle expressions of anger in body language, tone of voice, and/or facial expression; misinterpretation of anger (when it isn't there) is common. To avoid being overdiagnosed as angry, you can practice so that your face, body, and tone are less likely to be interpreted as angry. While anger can be a very effective emotion when used properly, the misreading of anger is generally detrimental. As anger is powerful and yet is often corrosive and destructive, we need to be judicious in recognizing and labeling anger correctly, and you benefit from having your own anger recognized and labeled correctly.

KEY TAKEAWAY

Just as context can affect interpretation of body language, mode of dress, and speech, there is always context around emotions. Context will help your accuracy in labeling emotions, including anger. Accurate perception of emotions is important data in pursuit of optimal doctor-patient connection.

PRACTICAL APPLICATIONS:
EMOTIONAL LOGIC

Draw a picture of five basic emotions

Feel each of five basic emotions and observe your face in the mirror as you feel them. Do this once a day for one week.

Next time you feel a strong emotion, name it, using the most precise label you possess (e.g., annoyance rather than anger).

Next time you feel sadness, and can name it, smile for 30 seconds (time yourself) and consciously think about how you are feeling changes.

Learn sign language, as this has been shown to aid perception of emotional facial expressions

In your next doctor-patient encounter, name one emotion you recognize.

Channel one emotion in a doctor-patient encounter to be more effective.

"It is very important to understand that emotional intelligence is not the opposite of intelligence, it is not the triumph of heart over head–it is the unique intersection of both."
— David Caruso, PhD, Psychologist

CORE AFFECT AND EMOTION CONSTRUCTION

Who you are, the language you speak, and your past experiences are all part of core affect, which has been proposed by Dr. Lisa Feldman Barrett as a neurobiologic basic for constructed emotion. Emotion is constructed by humans, and each human being might construct a different emotion based on their analysis of a given situation.

As an example, when my son was three and my daughter was six, we attended a three-week auditory oral program at John Tracy Center in Los Angeles. The first day of orientation, I was feeling hopeful but stressed. About fifteen families were there, and children were sent outside to play on the playground while parents shared a bit about themselves and their children. As I listened to the others and also gave a brief background on my son's diagnosis of auditory neuropathy and our journey with cochlear implants thus far, I began to tear up. As the session ended soon after I had shared our own personal experience, when my children reentered the room, my eyes and cheeks remained tear-stained.

My daughter's face mirrored my sadness and she hung back, seemingly reluctant to intrude into my space; during her kindergarten year, we had consciously learned about emotion, expression, and reactions. My son was (and remains) highly attuned to my emotional state, and through auditory verbal therapy, I had been exposing him to a near-constant narration of the world around us, including my thoughts, sensations, and reactions. When my son first saw my face, he let go of my daughter's hand and approached me, his face showing confusion. He came close to me and asked, "Why so sweaty?" as he touched my cheek. It struck me, in the moment, that I had not yet taught him the words "tears" or "cry" or "sad". His ability to properly construct my emotions and interpret the situation was somewhat hindered by his lack of language.

FURTHER READING

241 Naming emotions is helpful...Caruso DR, Rees LT. *A leader's guide to solving challenges with emotional intelligence.* Publishing Genius Press, 2018.

242 Five basic emotions...Ekman P. *Emotions Revealed.* New York: Times Books, 2013.

242 Certain facial expressions...Martinez A, Du S. How fast can we recognize facial expressions of emotion? *Vision Sciences Society Annual Meeting Abstract* 2010;10:607. AND Riess H, Kraft-Todd G. E.M.P.A.T.H.Y.: A tool to enhance nonverbal communication between clinicians and their patients. *Acad Med* 2014;89:1108–1112.

242 Emotions are also expressed in the body... Volynets S, et al. Bodily maps of emotions are culturally universal. *Emotion* 2019;doi:10.1037/ emo0000624.

244 Definitions of emotions, feelings, and moods... Caruso DR, Rees LT. *A leader's guide to solving challenges with emotional intelligence.* EI Press, 2018. AND Caruso D and Salovey P. *The Emotionally Intelligent Manager.* San Francisco: Jossey-Bass, 2004.

244 Emotions are culturally universal. Nummenmaa L, Glerean E, Hari R, Hietanen JK. Bodily maps of emotions. *PNAS* 2014;111:646-651.

246 Emotions come on quickly, are of relatively short duration...https://www.paulekman.com/ blog/mood-vs-emotion-difference-between-mood-emotion/

247 Visual processing of facial expressions... Martinez A, Du S. How fast can we recognize facial expressions of emotion? *Vision Sciences Society Annual Meeting Abstract* 2010;10:607. AND Schlegel K, Vicaria IM, Issacowitz DM, Hall JA. Effectiveness of a short audiovisual emotion recognition training program in adults. *Motiv Emot* 2017;4:646-660.

248 Microexpression training...https://www.paul-ekman.com/micro-expressions-training-tools/ AND Context is often important to correct interpretation of facial expressions...Heaven D. Why faces don't always tell the truth about feelings.nature.com/articles/d41586-020-0057-5

248 More recent research by Dr. Lisa Feldman Barrett...https://www.bostonmagazine.com/news/2013/06/25/emotions-facial-expressions-not-related/4/ AND Duncan S, Barrett LF. Affect is a form of cognition: A neurobiological analysis. *Cogn Emot* 2007;21:1184-1211.

249 Use logic to control your response...Caruso DR, Rees LT. *A leader's guide to solving challenges with emotional intelligence.* EI Skills Group Press, 2018.

250 "look up" how best to label your emotional state...https://www.ycei.org/ruler

252 Next time you feel sadness...Davis JI, Senghas A, Ochsner KN. How does facial feedback modulate emotional experience? *J Res Pers* 2009;43:822-829.

11 THE INTERPLAY OF WHAT YOU FEEL, HEAR, AND SEE

> "Do not learn how to react. Learn how to respond."
> — Buddha, Indian Philosopher and Religious Leader

As a toddler with two very expensive electronics perched somewhat precariously on his scalp and ears, my son would occasionally act out. One time when I was furious about something, and he was as well (he had just turned three, so had had cochlear implants for about one year) – he threw his electronic sound processors off his head. (*!! Tens of thousands of dollars of electronics flying through the air and crashing to the ground!!*) He knew I wanted him to keep them on. He knew the difference between them being on (hearing) and off (deafness) even then, glaring at me to do something about it. And I yelled, looking him straight in the eyes, "LISTEN!" There was no one to hear but me.

Even now, sound vs. silence is a constant, daily reminder – my son is deaf as soon as the external component comes off, whether momentarily, due to malfunction, deliberate removal, or at bedtime.

This is a reality that I don't mean to shy away from but I admit that it used to make me more uncomfortable, this silence that descends upon us and cannot be ignored. There are benefits – thunder and fireworks will not disturb his sleep; true and profound silence, which perhaps I could only experience in deep space, may be akin to nirvana – this latter is my hope. I have come to realize over time that his ability to turn sound on and off is powerful, something that I cannot do.

SELECTIVE PERCEPTION

Although my son achieved the goal of age-matched speech and language, he is still deaf. Increasingly, I see this as a unique strength that he has. When he wants to turn sound off, he can do so, actively and deliberately. Seeing him do this, I recognize that to a certain extent, I can do this as well. I see, hear, and feel every day. And I also don't see, don't hear, and don't feel certain things, either wantonly or inadvertently. My son is a daily reminder of this duality of perception that allows for self-determinism. My son will always have the dichotomy of hearing and deafness, and this ability is power.

When he has the sound processors off, divorced from auditory data, he can try to read lips or connect using people's facial expressions and body language. He is always reassured when I smile at him. Even with his sound processors on, as he is still mildly hearing impaired, especially in noisy situations, he also searches my face and body language for clues. Again, he tends to be cheered when I smile. When I have a neutral face or a disapproving face, he might get worried or might assume that he has done something wrong or I am unhappy. To avoid such misunderstandings on his part, I can control my facial expressions and ideally have a pleasant, or at least neutral, one. Cochlear implants and hearing give access to sound, but when my son chooses to go without sound, he is still the same person, and I can still communicate with him. His diagnosis of deafness is just one part of who he is. His world is not defined by deafness. He can adapt. He can choose to use his other senses.

Just as my son does, but perhaps less deliberately, we selectively use the perceptive modalities that are available to us. Based on what we focus on, the brain tends to group information from vision, hearing, and feeling into a cohesive story. Processing of facial expressions is not disconnected from speech but enhanced or suppressed depending on the congruency of speech and recognized emotion – you feel ease with harmony. You are biased toward synchrony. You avoid, or even ignore, discordant information. When a neutral face is paired with emotional speech, the face is read as emotional; even background music alters how a neutral face is interpreted. Context matters to the brain, on an almost automatic basis. Ultimately, the brain is looking for coherence in order to maximize efficiency – anything that makes the narrative jarring makes the brain work harder. Teaching the brain to appreciate concordance *and* search for discordance is practicing metaperception – thinking twice about what you see, hear, and feel.

FOR ME: THE INTERPLAY OF WHAT I SEE, HEAR, AND FEEL

Increased awareness of using emotional logic while creating observing and listening habits has helped me immensely in my relationship with not only my son but also my patients, colleagues, and those whom I teach. Visual, auditory, and emotional perception aid my interactions with patients, colleagues and other medical professionals, as well as my children's teachers, staff, and my own mentors. Through double checking initial, fast perceptions with slower, more careful analysis, I can communicate better and practice medicine more fully. It is also helpful to prepare ahead of time, and there are particular catchphrases that doctors and patients can use for better communication (see **Chapter 4**).

As quickly as possible, name the ink color of the following words:

BOX
GATE
DEAR
COMB

HATE
DEAD
POX
BOMB

For many people, the second group of words takes a bit longer. This exercise is an example of the *emotional* Stroop effect. The Stroop effect (see **Chapter 3**) demonstrates that naming colors is made more difficult by distracting the brain with the action of reading. The emotional Stroop effect is a result of mixing in words that have associated emotion (e.g. dead, bomb) with words that are neutral (e.g. dear, comb). Color processing tends to be delayed for "negative" words like "cancer" or "war" compared to neutral words like "clock". In other words, a negative emotional reaction from a word is encoded first, using up brain power and slowing down visual recognition. Emotional data takes primacy, prior to visual identification of simple colors.

Because the brain predictably encodes emotions first, it is useful to polish your skills in correctly identifying emotion in facial expressions, body language, and vocalizations in a doctor-patient encounter. The initial, rapid processing of emotion greatly determines how you subsequently interpret what you see and hear. Much as wearing tinted sunglasses will brighten or darken everything around you, emotion data overlays your perceptions.

64OR-PATIENT CONNECTION

DOCTOR-PATIENT CONNECTION: THE INTERPLAY OF SEEING, HEARING, FEELING

Being aware of neural processing will help you in healthcare encounters – you will recognize emotions more readily and be able to use emotional logic to respond in the most appropriate fashion. Knowing that the primacy of emotional reactions may control what is subsequently seen or heard, you can pause, you can monitor body language, and you can carefully listen to what is said aloud. The more you do this, the more it will become habit, in daily life as well as in doctor-patient interactions.

KEY TAKEAWAY

Dr. Rana Awdish, a doctor who ultimately recovered from multi-organ failure and near death, writes, "Medicine cannot heal in a vacuum; it requires connection." To create connection, you can form habits of observing, listening, and emotional logic. Important data to collect include what you see of body language, what you hear from language and tone of voice, and what you understand doctors and patients as feeling in a given interaction. As you become more adept with your observations, listening ability, and emotional logic, you will more skillfully pilot

"The goal is to turn data into information and information into insight."
—Carly Fiorina, Former CEO, Hewlett Packard

important healthcare relationships, avoid detrimental crash landings, and guide reliable doctor-patient connection.

Dr. Viktor E. Frankl, renowned psychiatrist and author of *Man's Search for Meaning,* wrote that for half a century, "psychiatry tried to interpret the human mind merely as a mechanism, and consequently the therapy of mental disease merely in terms of technique." He suggested, "A doctor, however, who would still interpret his own role mainly as that of a technician would confess that he sees in his patient nothing more than a machine, instead of seeing the human being behind the disease!"

Mind and body are surely more than mechanisms, doctors are not only technicians, and patients are definitely not machines. It is through doctor-patient connection that people will remain in sight. Disease must allow, rather than prevent, a space to acknowledge and bear witness to the depth of humanity.

PRACTICAL APPLICATIONS: OBSERVE, LISTEN, AND USE EMOTIONAL LOGIC

Imagine a difficult doctor-patient conversation, including body language, speech, and emotions (facial expressions, voice prosody) if the interaction is going well versus if the interaction is going poorly.

After experiencing a difficult conversation between doctor and patient, think back on body language, speech, and emotions (facial expressions, voice prosody). Try to remember if spoken words were congruent with what you saw, felt, and heard. For whatever you recall, consider how aware you were of it in the moment and if you were able to use that data as you responded.

Each doctor-patient interaction, note one thing about body language, speech, or emotions, and consider how that influenced you.

Each doctor-patient interaction, consider the primacy of emotions and try to note at least one expressed emotion by doctor or patient.

FURTHER READING

260 When a neutral face is paired with emotional speech…Schirmer A, et al. Emotion perception from face, voice, and touch: Comparisons and convergence. *Trends Cogn Sci* 2017;21:216-228. AND Klasen M, et al. Multisensory emotions: perception, combination and underlying neural processes. *Rev Neurosci* 2012;23:381-392.

260 Background music alters how a neutral face… Woloszyn MR, Ewert L. Memory for facial expression is influenced by the background music playing during study. *Adv Cogn Psychol* 2012;8:226-233. AND Logeswaran, N. & Bhattacharya, J. Crossmodal transfer of emotion by music. *Neurosci Lett* 2009;455:129-133.

263 The *emotional* Stroop effect…Ben-Haim MS, et al. The emotional Stroop task: Assessing cognitive performance under exposure to emotional content. *J Vis Exp* 2016;112;53720.

264 "Medicine cannot heal in a vacuum; it requires connection."…Awdish R. *In Shock: My Journey from Death to Recovery and the Redemptive Power of Hope.* St Martin's Press, 2017.

265 Dr. Viktor E. Frankl, renowned psychiatrist and author of *Man's Search for Meaning,* writes that for half a century…Frankl, VE. *Man's Search for Meaning.* Boston: Beacon Press, 2014, page 152.

APPENDIX

MINDSET

Growth Mindset	Fixed Mindset
Improvement happens with work	Talent and smarts are fixed and unchangeable
Challenges help you improve	Challenges mean you aren't good enough
Hard work/effort means you are learning	Effort means you are out of your league
Things should feel hard	Things should feel easy
Failing shows you can improve	Failing means you are a failure
Challenges are sought out	Challenges are avoided

EXAMPLES OF COGNITIVE BIAS

ANCHORING

Tendency to rely too much on one piece of information, especially what is initially learned

Healthcare Example

My son's newborn hearing test (termed otoacoustic emissions testing [OAE]) was normal, and medical professionals disregarded that there are rare causes of deafness with normal OAE

Life Example

Women are underrepresented in all positions of power, and children "learn" early on that men are more likely to be heads of companies, businesses, and countries. As children grow up, this implicit bias has stayed with many men and women, and men are more likely to be hired for a given position than women with identical qualifications.

ATTENTIONAL

Tendency to notice only certain things

Healthcare Example

Early on when first looking at microscopic slides of skin, medical students tend to see the ink around the tissue (placed there during processing of the tissue), ignoring the tumor within the tissue. You tend to notice what is most familiar.

Life Example

Before I began drawing using a book by Betty Edwards, I would notice the shapes of objects around me rather than the empty space in between objects. After doing several drawings focused on the negative space – the angles and shapes around and between perceived figures – now when I look up at the sky through the trees, I am more able to see the shape of the sky between the leaves and not just the leaves.

AUTHORITY

Tendency to trust those in authority

Healthcare Example

I trusted the medical professionals that told me my son had normal hearing, despite my instinct

Life Example

The COVID-19 pandemic was handled very differently by different countries, often based on the authority of governments and what was recommended by authority figures and mandated by law.

AVAILABILITY

Tendency to use information that you can recall easily

Healthcare Example

Before I started college, I had a bout of extreme abdominal pain of unclear etiology. It was so bad that I went to the emergency room. The doctor there asked me repeatedly if I could be pregnant, despite my telling him there was no chance. The doctor was hyperfocused on teenage pregnancy because it is common and because young patients are often aware of but unable to admit to pregnancy.

CONFIRMATION

Searching for evidence that supports something already "known" or "believed to be true" and ignoring what doesn't fit.

Healthcare and Life Example

Early on in the COVID-19 pandemic, people had wide-ranging opinions on the risk of SARS-CoV-2 transmission in the community based on what information they were exposed to and chose to read.

Life Example

I read something in the news and then I hear someone say it, and I believe it to be true.

MORE ABOUT AUDITORY VERBAL THERAPY (AVT)

AVT has 10 principles that help to create a listening habit. Initial, early diagnosis of hearing loss is key, and much effort and work could be avoided by diagnosis and intervention during the newborn to six-month period (my son's late diagnosis precluded this type of easier acquisition of language). Verbal language can be learned by anyone with effective auditory access (hearing), and the earlier that infants get that access, chances are higher of avoiding speech and language delays.

With any delay in access to sound, speech, and spoken language may not develop naturally without active intervention. AVT is a method of activating habitual, conscious language development, and clear, defined goals are key to monitoring effective progress. Measurable goals are necessary to document effectiveness of interventions (examples below).

PRINCIPLES OF AUDITORY VERBAL THERAPY (AVT)*

Immediately:

1. *Diagnose hearing loss as early as possible, followed by audiologic management and AVT.*

2. *Use appropriate, state-of-the-art hearing technology.*

Guide and coach parents to help their child:

3. *Use hearing as the primary sensory modality in developing listening and spoken language.*

4. *By becoming the primary facilitators of their child's listening and spoken language development through active, consistent participation in individualized AVT.*

5. *By creating environments that support listening for the acquisition of spoken language throughout the child's daily activities.*

6. *Integrate listening and spoken language into all aspects of the child's life.*

7. *By using natural developmental patterns of audition, speech, language, cognition, and communication.*

8. *Self-monitor spoken language through listening.*

Long-term:

9. *Administer formal and informal diagnostic assessments to develop individualized auditory verbal treatment plans, to monitor progress and to evaluate the effectiveness of the plans for the child and family.*

10. *Promote education in regular schools with peers who have typical hearing and with appropriate services.*

*Adapted from AG Bell, https://agbellacademy.org/certification/principles-of-lsl-specialists/

It is important to keep in mind that there are many factors that affect spoken language development, for example: the age of diagnosis of hearing loss/deafness, the age of receiving working hearing aids or cochlear implants, the age that early intervention starts, pre-existing teacher and parent expectations, and what approach is used for language development.

MEASURABLE GOALS – EXAMPLES FOR MY SON AT AGE THREE

☐ Emphasize 2-word combinations. Highlight the "s" in plural words and the final strong sound to call attention to the end of words.

☐ Practice babbling – dance while saying the sounds.

☐ Pause during conversation to give him a chance to initiate.

☐ When he holds an object and looks at you, let him say something before you do.

☐ Repeat 4-5-word sentences with known vocabulary 90% of the time and 6-7-word sentences with known vocabulary 80% of the time.

☐ Follow simple directions showing understanding of in/on/under 85% of the time and commands containing 2 critical attributes 85% of the time.

☐ Answer simple "what happened" questions 85% of the time, "who is (verb)ing" questions 85% of the time, and "what is (agent) doing" questions 80% of the time.

☐ Show understanding of singular and plural in commands 80% of the time.

☐ Take 2 turns in conversation with adults without prompts 85% of the time and 4-5 turns in conversation with adults without prompts 80% of the time.

LINGUISTIC ASPECTS OF CHARISMA AND PRESENCE*

Tier 1: Key aspects to be aware of

Simplification
Speed control~
Energy
Priming

Tier 2: Secondary aspects to work on

The last idea
Gestures
Emotion words, spoken aloud

Tier 3: Tertiary aspects to focus on

Mirroring
Framing
Humanized statistics

SKILL AREAS OF SPEECH*

Fluency
Organization
Charisma
Vocabulary
Pronunciation
Cognition
Cohesion
Strategy
Word choices
Grammar

---

*Adapted from William Vance, PhD, linguist and director of Executive Voice
~Note that you can read faster than you can speak (about 500 words/ minute), while speech is generally about 100-200 words/minute

A LINGUISTIC REPORT

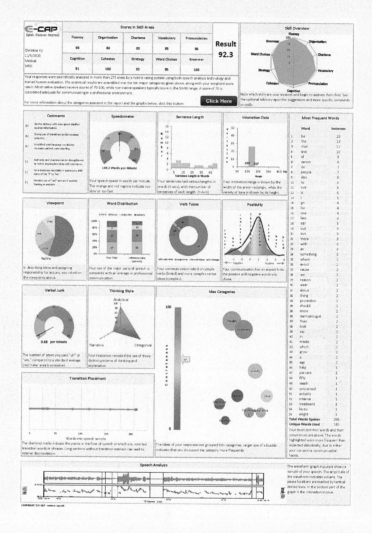

METACOGNITION AND EMOTIONS*

Gut feeling – "emotions are bad"	Analyzed feeling – "emotions are helpful"
Don't get too excited	*Get excited*
You're too emotional	*Get emotional*
Be rational	*Be emotional, but logically so*

EMOTIONAL INTELLIGENCE*

Map *How do I/we feel?*	Become aware of emotions (yours and others) – be able to identify them and know how they are expressed
Match *How does it influence what I/we think/do?*	Match others' emotions to connect. Match the emotion to the task
Meaning *Why do I/we feel this way? How did it/can it change?*	Understand the underlying meaning and causes of feelings – use affective forecasting and realize emotions are dynamic
Move *How can I use this feeling to motivate me and others?*	Manage emotions to be more effective and influence others productively

*Adapted from Caruso and Salovey, *The Emotionally Intelligent Manager* and Caruso and Rees, *A Leader's Guide to Solving Challenges wit*

MORE ABOUT EMOTIONS

Trigger	Range (least intense to most intense)	Vocalization	Body
Anger			
Someone else's anger Not getting your way Unfairness Betrayal Rejection	Annoyance Argumenta- tiveness Fury	Raised voice Sharp edge to words	Flushing Sweating Leaning forward Expanding chest Clenching jaw or hands Tensing muscles
Contempt			
Dislike for and feeling superi-or to another person or group		Disapproving sounds Smug tone	Can be similar to anger or happi- ness Gazing down- ward along the nose Rolling eyes
Disgust			
Something or someone offensive	Dislike Repugnance Abhorrence	"Yuck", "Ew" Choking Gagging	Nausea Turning head away Hunching over
Joy (enjoyment, happiness)*			
Sensory pleasure Human goodness Humor Human connection Beauty Achievement	Sensory plea- sure Excitement Ecstasy	Sigh Squeal Exclamation Giggling Laughter	Lightness Energy Comforting warmth Tingling Groundedness Upright or re- laxed posture

Fear

Threat of harm	Trepidation	Higher pitch	Coldness
	Nervousness	Strained tone	Trouble breath-ing
	Anxiety	Screaming	Sweating
	Desperation		Trembling
	Panic		Tight arms/legs
	Horror		Posture frozen or moving away
	Terror		

Sadness

Loss	Disappoint-ment	Lower or softer pitch	Tight chest
	Discourage-ment	-or-	Heavy limbs
	Resignation	Higher and louder pitch	Watery eyes
	Helplessness	Sobs	Stinging throat
	Despair	Heaving	Posture weak
	Grief	Quavering	Face turned away
	Anguish		

Surprise^

Sudden and/ or unexpected event		Gasp	Attentiveness
			Moving hands up
			Recoiling

*As a feeling, rather than a state of well-being

^Briefest emotion

INDEX